FLUSH YOUR FAT 4GOOD

Be Lean and Healthy for Life!

JACKIE PADGETTE-BAIRD
DR. VICTORIA C. ARCADI
KATHLEEN J. POWELL

Waterside Press

Printed in the United States of America

ISBN-13: 978-0-9627145-6-6 print edition
ISBN-13: 978-1-943625-97-0 ebook edition

Waterside Publishing
2055 Oxford Ave
Cardiff, CA 92007
www.waterside.com

To Jennifer Powell

One of the most inspiring metamorphoses through Flush Your Fat 4Good has been Jennifer Powell. In ten months, Jennifer not only lost 120 inches and 92 pounds but became a Coach and host of our Power100 Heroes support call. She awakened herself and faced her paradigms that had kept her hostage in an obese body for over thirty years. Flying free like a butterfly in life without the fear of going backwards again and again has transformed Jennifer into one of the most admired FYF4Good Buddies.

We have a huge amount of gratitude for Jennifer's courage to change her life, her compassion to help others embrace this journey, her devotion to do whatever is needed to help us bring FYF4Good to the world, and for all the late nights of research, reading, and editing this book to make sure we did not miss anything.

We love you, Coach Jennifer Powell!

"In **Flush Your Fat 4Good**, the authors have done an amazing job of directly helping people who are looking to get healthy and transform their lives. Their authentic journey, not about being on a diet, but changing their Lifestyle is one that all of us can learn from. **Read it. Share it!**"

Kara Goldin
Founder & CEO HINT, INC.

"I lost 2 of my best friends to health problems associated with obesity. One was just 40 years old and died of a heart attack while sleeping in bed. I want to help as many people as I can by motivating them to improve on what they eat, the supplements they take, and the exercises they do. Diets may provide temporary weight loss, but changing one's lifestyle is a must to maintain permanent results. **Flush Your Fat 4Good** provides the best possible way. I hope that my recommendations for adhering to the ideas described will encourage you to read and follow what is laid out in a simple, understandable, and truthful manner in this "Lifestyle" changing book."

Don "The Dragon" Wilson
11 Time Professional Kickboxing World Champion
European Marital Arts Hall of Famer
Action Film Actor

"We are never too old to learn how to improve our lives. This book is a great inspirational blueprint for getting lean and healthy **4Good!**"

Esther Wojcicki
Founder GlobalMoonshots.org
Founder Palo Alto High Media Arts Program

"As a doctor of holistic medicine, my first line of defense is always nutrition. But I don't generally promote "diets" because the first 3 letters of the word DIET are DIE! Diets are short term fixes, tend to be radical, far from healthy, and don't constitute lifestyle change! A lifestyle change is the only path to follow if you're looking for a healthy, long life! **Flush Your Fat 4Good** is just that. The authors have laid out a journey for all kinds of diet preferences (I am a vegan) in order to reach your goals **4GOOD!**"

Dr. Spice Williams-Crosby, MFS, MS, PhD
Actress / Stuntwoman / Martial Artist

"One need only look around at young and old to see that obesity is a huge global problem. So what are you going to do to tackle this problem if you are obese or members of your family are? My advice is to obtain and digest a copy of this extremely readable book that gives you comprehensive advice based on many years of the authors' experience in the field. It also offers an excellent support system that is always available."

Robert K. Murray
Emeritus Professor of Biochemistry

"This is a great book for those that are tired of being over fat and want a healthy way to lean down and stay that way. No matter what your eating preferences (I am a vegan), the base principles behind this valuable system might just be the answer for you. Great job guys!"

Gregory Crosby
Writer / Producer "Hacksaw Ridge"

"Positive change is preceded by a decision. Change happens from the inside out; it starts with our thinking. If you want to change your health or your weight, it's a matter of making an irrevocable decision to do things differently. **FLUSH YOUR FAT 4GOOD** is a wonderful guide to making the lasting change you seek. Use your marvelous imagination and build a beautiful image of a healthier, leaner you. Make a decision today!"

Bob Proctor
Master Success Coach
Teacher in The Secret

"I have lived the FYF4Good Phase 2 Lifestyle for some time and it has had a profound effect on my health, energy, digestion, and physical capacity. This book gives you a way to live that is sustainable, easy-to-understand, and *evolved*."

Halfdan Hussey
Co-Founder & CEO
Cinequest

CONTENTS

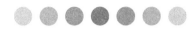

FYF4Good Lifestyle Phase 1: Eating and Nutrifying to Lose the Fat

FYF4Good Lifestyle Phase 2: Eating and Nutrifying

Traveling, Special Grocery Shopping, Eating Out, and Holidays

Globesity

FYF4Good Power100 Heroes

ACKNOWLEDGMENTS

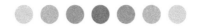

We want to give thanks and acknowledgment to those that have inspired, encouraged and strongly requested us to write this book.

- ❖ Through divine intervention, this Lifestyle, was given to not only Jackie but to the world. Therefore our gracious gratitude goes to God as our lives are now lean, healthier, and happy 4Good. We are now honored to help others change their lives for the better.

- ❖ To Bob Proctor and Sandy Gallagher for inspiring us to dream beyond all we thought was possible and to know that it is already real.

- ❖ We are so grateful and thankful to our thousands of FYF4Good Buddies and especially to our Power100 Heroes who have given life a second chance with Flush Your Fat 4Good.

- ❖ We would like to thank William Gladstone, our literary agent, who we believe came to us through the Law of Attraction as we prayed at 11:11 every day for an agent that could understand and see the global benefit of Flush Your Fat 4Good.

- ❖ To our amazing editor, Nancy Sugihara. We will miss your 2:00 a.m. emails and incredible kindness. You taught us so much.

- ❖ And finally … We thank Dr. R.K. Murray for reading the manuscript and for making helpful suggestions.

A NOTE TO READERS ABOUT STARTING

THE FLUSH YOUR FAT 4GOOD LIFESTYLE

Always consult your health care practitioner before making drastic changes to your lifestyle. When you change the way you eat, the supplements you put into your body, and the physical activity you do daily, your body will start to change. And if you are like most of us living the Flush Your Fat 4Good (FYF4Good) Lifestyle, your body will start to change very quickly. If you are on medications or have been diagnosed with ailments or medical conditions, you want your physician to know what you are doing so they can monitor you and make modifications to your treatment plan. Countless people living the FYF4Good Lifestyle have seen huge health benefits and have been able to reduce, and in many cases, eliminate medications they were prescribed for years. This must be done by, and with, your health care practitioner's approval, direction, and monitoring.

It is mandatory that people who have been diagnosed with liver or kidney disease consult with their health care practitioner for approval before starting this Lifestyle. Both liver and kidney disease can be very serious and at worst, life-threatening. These conditions require constant monitoring by your health care practitioner. Therefore, this information would need to be put into your medical chart so you can be monitored effectively.

If you have had a recent heart attack you must consult your health care practitioner before starting. The heart is a critical organ in the body. After a serious traumatic event such as a heart attack, you are going to be compromised, weak, fragile, vulnerable, and very unstable. You probably have been prescribed medications to aid stability of your body and healing and recovery. Be sure to have your health care practitioner review FYF4Good before beginning the Lifestyle recommendations to make sure it will be appropriate to your situation.

If you are pregnant or lactating, consult with your midwife or OB/GYN before beginning FYF4Good. Phase 1 may be appropriate for a short duration, but it is advised that you are under your health care practitioner's supervision. Phase 2 is for a *Lifetime* and has been shown to be appropriate during pregnancy. But once again, it is advised that you consult your practitioner in charge of your pregnancy and together review FYF4Good Phase 2 before starting. Once the baby is born, mothers can continue to follow Phase 2, and then after the baby is weaned from the breast milk, mothers can begin with Phase 1 to effectively and rapidly get that pregnancy fat off. Once again, run all of this by your midwife, OB/GYN or health care practitioner in charge of your birth.

Since the FYF4Good Lifestyle is all about digestion, absorption, and elimination, it can be very beneficial during pregnancy because digestion can be less than optimal due to stresses, as well as anatomical and physiological changes that are constantly occurring all through gestation. Digestion is particularly affected because gastric emptying is slowed, and digestive juices can be less than optimum due to the rise of progesterone levels during pregnancy. Additionally, elimination of sugar, cow dairy products, and excessive starches can help to benefit and maintain a healthier pregnancy, birth, and recovery. *You Can Never Go Wrong Eating Right!* Especially when eating for two! With the proper food and nutritional supplement recommendations, healthy babies have been delivered with less excessive maternal weight gain as well as fewer complications and impressive recoveries.

This Lifestyle is not a diet. It is not a fad. It is not a quick fix. It will be evident and very obvious to you when your digestive system returns to optimal function, something the majority of overfat people have not experienced in years. FYF4Good is not something that you will ever want to stop because you will feel such an improved sense of well-being!

INTRODUCTION

WHAT IS FLUSH YOUR FAT 4GOOD?

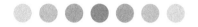

All that you thought it was, it's NOT!

If you are like most people, your brain has been on unaware autopilot about the subjects of *food* and your *body* for a very long time. It needs to wake up and think in a brand-new way, a *Lifestyle* way. And here is how it can happen. Welcome to Flush Your Fat 4Good (FYF4Good). This is not a "diet." This is not a "plan" or a "fad." FYF4Good is a *Lifestyle* unlike anything you have ever known before.

Throw out everything you know about eating, dieting, and exercising. This includes the Food Pyramid from grade school, the four basic food groups, counting calories on the latest fad diet, adding up points, starving yourself, or believing the only way to lose weight is hard-core cardio exercising... Get rid of this, NOW! Everything you learned from your parents and relatives or read in a diet book. All of it!

Then open your mind. You are the one in charge and will know exactly what you need to do. You are beginning a journey to a new, leaner, healthier, in control *you*!

You now have in your hands perhaps the most important book you will ever read in your life. You will learn how to feed and nutrify your body as the engine to rapidly burn the fat, and we mean rapid! Women can expect to lose about ten to twelve pounds of fat and men about twelve to fifteen pounds of fat, per month.

With this new Lifestyle, you will literally eat your way to health. Your body will become lean, while maintaining the integrity of your bones, blood, tissue, muscles, and organs. Moreover, by eliminating the stress on your body from carrying extra fat, and by properly feeding and nutrifying your body, your hormones will balance, your digestive system will start to work correctly, and you will be on the road to optimal health.

Better still, FYF4Good is not hard! It is different, but not difficult. In fact many FYF4Good Buddies say it is *easy*! If you are committed to following the FYF4Good *Lifestyle to a "T"* your body will become trim and healthy in an amazingly short period of time. And it will last. You will maintain your new you for a lifetime.

At FYF4Good there is a support team to answer questions, as well as encourage you. You will learn what to do, for the rest of your life, to make sure you never struggle with unnecessary fat again. Think about how you learned to ride a bike or drive a stick shift car. At first seemed a little awkward, right? But once you got it down, you never forgot, it became second nature, a part of your life. Well, it is the same with FYF4Good, which is *A Lifestyle for a Lifetime!* It will become an invaluable part of you. And the best part: FYF4Good is fun!

Let us say it again. FYF4Good is *A Lifestyle for a Lifetime!* It is not a "diet." Diets do not work, and there is so much research out there that is easy to access on the internet that shows this. FYF4Good is not a "diet." It is not something to do for three months before you go on vacation, or get married or head to your class reunion. FYF4Good is *A Lifestyle for a Lifetime!* To fully grasp what that means, we should take a look at why diets don't work.

WHY DIETS DON'T WORK!
Understand this, before it is too late

In the United States alone there are over forty-five million people on a diet on any given day. *Forty-Five Million People!*

There are diets that reduce carbohydrates, restrict calories, restrict portions, include only protein, are vegetarian, or Mediterranean—the list goes on. There are diets that require fasting or make us drink our food. Diets that have us eat like ancient humans. Diets can be approached by category: Macrobiotic, Vegan, Omnivorous, Carnivorous, Fruitarian, Paleolithic, Lacto-Ovo-Vegetarian … *Say what?* If you search on the internet for "list of diets," you will find directories of over six hundred weight-loss diets. *Over Six Hundred!*

The diet industry is over *Sixty-Six Billion Dollars* and growing! That is a lot of books, a lot of shakes and bars, a lot of pills, a lot of weight-loss centers, and a lot of prepackaged food! If any one of these six hundred-plus diets "worked," it would have risen to the top a long time ago. And … there is a really good reason *why* they do not want you to be successful at dieting. Think of all the money they would lose!

And guess what? If you are one that has experienced painful yo-yo dieting, you should not think that putting that fat back on your body is your fault. It is not about your lack of willpower or self-control. In fact your willpower and self-control are exercised daily when dieting. It goes much deeper than that.

Let's take a look at what happens when you "go on a diet."

First of all, our bodies were not made to "need to" diet. You should eat in a healthy way every day, eating properly, and eating enough to sustain your body with energy and nutrition for strength, regulation, and protection.

The Biological Impact of Dieting

There are three major sets of biological effects on our body when we diet: neurological, hormonal, and metabolic:

> The **Neurological Effects** are almost immediate. Being deprived of foods that are addicting drives people nuts. It makes them irritable, angry, short tempered, sad, and moody. When we place restrictions on our food, our brain becomes overly responsive to it. For many it is the same as what a drug addict goes through. "There is the food! I see it! Can I eat it now? I want that!" Because our brain starts to focus on it, it becomes one of the most important topics in our brain. With the number one question all through the day, "When am I going to eat next?"!

The **Hormonal Effects** are ones we may not realize are happening, and they can be very damaging. Our bodies were designed in a way that if food supplies are restricted, our body will become "stressed" thinking it is beginning to starve. The body then will start producing high levels of cortisol. And guess what this hormone does? It slows down the rate at which our body burns calories and we start to store FAT. The body has one goal: TO SURVIVE! In other words, your body thinks it might be going down and puts on reserves to sustain your life. So when you reduce the number of calories you are consuming, your body will start conserving. Diets that focus on calorie counting and restriction, portion control, or fasting are all very stressful and may actually do harm to the body. While you might have short-term results on the scale (coming from water loss and muscle and bone breakdown) your body fat could have very likely gone UP! And the more times you do this, the harder it is on the body. Many diets for weight loss have shown that participants lose as much as 50 percent of fat and 50 percent bone and muscle. When you gain your fat back, you do not gain the corresponding muscle with it. Each time you go back on a diet, you lose a little more of the muscle and bone structure that support your body. This cycle leads to a higher percentage of body fat.

The **Metabolic Effects** can be seen on the scale. If calories are restricted, our body will figure out a way to survive on fewer calories. Your metabolism will slow down, so your weight loss will also slow down. The body does not know what you have planned for dinner, or tomorrow, or next week. All it knows is that it is getting less, the supply chain is shutting down, and it needs to run on less! This has been very damaging for those in weight-loss contests and on weight-loss competition reality TV shows.

The Mental Impact of Dieting

This is different from the neurological effects. Being hungry most of the time is common when dieting. A diet has rules: eat this, do not eat that, count to this number and stop, measure this. But we never learn WHY we should eat this and not that. Diets rarely teach us what the actual nutrients are in the food, which is important for the health of our body. Diets almost never focus on or mention getting our digestive system to work correctly so we can absorb the nutrients from the foods we eat. They do not give us the knowledge we need to make the right choices. And they almost never help us evolve our relationship with food. How do we look at food? Will it taste good? Is it just fuel to survive? Do we look at desserts as a "treat" or "reward"? Do we have "comfort food"? What food will "make us feel better"?

Long-term success after dieting has a high failure rate because we never learned WHAT we should be eating, WHY we should be eating it, HOW we should eat and how we should FEEL about it! Knowledge is power! The ingredients in many of the "diet foods" and the effects they have on our body are frightening.

When we are addicted to the foods that we know could hurt us, to recognize this would be the first step to changing this paradigm and insure success 4Good. The relationship you have with your foods, mentally, should be one of respect, harmony, balance, healing and admiration. Anything that goes into your mouth should build, repair, and maintain the integrity of your bones, blood, tissue, muscles, and organs. If your self-respect and self-esteem are healthy, you want foods that are "good" for you. This of course assumes you are educated about healthy foods. Everyone knows something about bad foods, and many people say, "It is okay, just in moderation"! This parallels the behavior of the victim with Stockholm Food Syndrome. Even when you know it is hurting you, you are compelled to eat it anyway. That is how you live only a moderate life—remaining a victim of your foods and not living an Optimal Life! And the moderate life leads to a sicker life as time goes by. This soon becomes a downward spiral out of control.

It is all about the "Mindset." The mental level on which we vibrate will become a magnet to whatever you feel about yourself on that level. To want to feel lean and healthy, happy and vibrant, means you *must* choose the right foods for your body. The "*Healthy Body, Healthy Mind*" level: a Mindset of desiring "*The Optimal Health Level*" regardless of your circumstances. FYF4Good is your ticket to a new life of freedom! Within days of starting FYF4Good, your energy will start to vibrate in a way that you may not have felt for a long time, if ever. There is a cleanliness feeling, a positive feeling, a stronger feeling of body and self, a sense of control. The happy vibe is created by the cleaner body. Maintaining the FYF4Good Lifestyle for at least four to six months (the life of a red blood cell is four months) starts to solidify the Paradigm Shift of your relationship with your foods. Thus, *A Lifestyle for a Lifetime* has begun.

The Lack of "Fun" When Dieting

Have you ever heard anyone talk about how much FUN dieting is? Of course not. Almost all dieting is about restriction, always being hungry, cravings and struggles with will-power, mood swings, deprivation, and just grinding it out. This brings stress and tension (open the cortisol flood gates)! Most people that have "gone on a diet" step on the scale every day, sometimes multiple times a day. *Did I win today? I should not have eaten that extra egg. Why did I drink that extra glass of water?* It is almost never about: *How do you feel? Are you having any satisfaction? Why are you doing this?*

There are some other really bad things about many of the diets that are out there besides the biological, mental, and lack-of-fun effects on your body. Let's talk about *toxins*. Just because something is claimed to be "healthy" or to provide "essential vitamins and minerals" does not mean it is a good choice. Think about the following:

- Prepackaged Foods: These are full of preservatives and/or chemicals to greatly extend their shelf life, sometimes for years, but are they real food anymore? The body often cannot recognize what to do with them. Therefore, whatever little nutrition may have been in the food they were made from is not recognized or absorbed by the body.
- Synthetic Supplements: There is a whole section in this book and a lot of research online as to why it is not beneficial in most cases to take synthetic supplements. They are loosely regulated and made in a lab. Most contain coal tar, petroleum, petroleum by-products, ground-up rocks, iron shavings and/or chemicals, which our bodies cannot recognize. Synthetic supplements are not absorbed well

because our bodies were designed to only recognize real food. The body has to expend energy to try to figure out what to do with these non-food substances. Many times, the body robs Peter to pay Paul, and other deficiencies are created in an effort to absorb them.

• Meal Replacement Shakes: Here are several facts about meal replacement shakes.

The vitamins and minerals are synthetic in most shakes.

Most contain added sugar/sweeteners: Which keeps the craving going as sugar acts like *cocaine on the brain!*

They may contain artificial ingredients (thickeners, preservatives, color, flavorings).

They are designed as meal replacements, which is simply a calorie restriction philosophy that decreases the metabolism, so that when one returns to regular food with a normal calorie intake, weight gain is inevitable.

They can cause digestive issues such as indigestion, heartburn, constipation, and bloating.

Most are low in protein and fiber designed to make you feel full, but from what?

The research is scarce and not conclusive showing meal replacement shakes provide a means for lasting weight loss or weight maintenance.

Digestion starts in the mouth when you chew or masticate your food. Saliva is produced, and your stomach is notified to get those digestive enzymes ready. Chewing increases the surface area of the food to allow more efficient break down by your digestive enzymes. As chewing continues, the food is made softer and warmer, and the digestive enzymes in saliva begin to break down carbohydrates in the food. After chewing, the food is swallowed. This chewed food, known as the bolus of food, enters the esophagus via peristalsis (wavelike movement that continues throughout the digestive tube propelling food through) and continues on to the stomach, where the next step of digestion occurs.

If you drink your food, it will bypass the first process of your digestive system, mastication (chewing). The stomach will have to figure out what to do with the drink when it arrives. There will be minimal and rapid absorption of the few nutrients contained in the drink because it is liquid. The best way to absorb nutrients is through a reasonable transit time, which is missing in this case. Eating solid food allows for slow absorption as the bolus of food hits the stomach and the body begins to secrete the digestive enzymes to break it down. After the breakdown in the stomach, fiber and broken-down nutrients continue into and through the twenty feet (six meters) of small intestine. This is where most of the nutrients are absorbed into the body. It would stand to reason that since the small intestine is that long, it is designed to absorb food gradually and slowly as peristalsis carries it through to the colon.

When drinking liquid meals, most of the digestive processes and duties of the body are eliminated or minimized dramatically because the food is liquid. Therefore, laxity of the digestive system may result. If you don't use it, you lose it! Newborns have to drink their food, in the form of breast milk, but only until they get teeth. The teeth signify the formation and ability of their bodies to make and release digestive enzymes. Cutting teeth is when babies are now supposed to be given whole foods to add to their nutrition. So why would adults want to drink their food like a newborn baby?

- Meal Replacement Bars and Snacks: While meal replacement bars and snacks may help you keep your blood sugar up between meals, they often contain added sugar to make them taste good like a cookie, candy bar, or some other sweet treat. An insulin spike will be triggered from the high sugar content, usually followed by a sharp drop in blood sugar. It is a sweet starchy treat that is not fresh, has no fluids, and contains preservatives that will allow it to sit on a shelf for a very long period of time … sometimes years. What do you think happens when you put those preservatives in your body? Preservatives are chemicals that the body treats as toxins. The body does not know how to process them, so they hinder the digestive system. They get stored in fat cells and ultimately will have to be processed by the liver. There are a few bars that are clean of toxins, but it is still difficult for the body to process them.

There are no fluids or freshness in these bars. They will slow down the digestion. If you are stuck on a deserted island or out camping without the means to eat fresh food, they would come in handy until you are rescued or return home to feed yourself appropriately! But if you choose to eat these every day, the negative effect on your body is certain.

So let us say it one more time! **FYF4Good is NOT a diet. It is _A Lifestyle for a Lifetime!_** You will have all the knowledge and all the power to lose the fat, keep it off for the rest of your life, _and_ eat and nutrify your body for optimal health! So keep reading. What do you have to lose?

CHANGING THE MIND

For any change to be truly permanent, it must not be just in the body; it also must occur in the mind. Unfortunately many of us have inherited a false "paradigm" about _everything_ we know about food. We routinely eat certain foods because our family did. Habits and behaviors were passed down to us from our ancestors. For example, if we got hurt or were upset as a child, food or sweet treats were often provided to "make us feel better" or help us stop crying. Most people live unconsciously, and do not stop to consider that offering this might lead to creating bad habits in that child. If you are thinking "emotional eating," you are right on the money. These mind patterns, imprinted on us at such an early age, have, in part, prevented healthy choices being made during stressful times. Not only are _we_ affected; there is also a significant, trickle-down impact on close family members and loved ones.

To drive genuine, lasting change, one really needs to understand how the mind works. The human mind can be broken down into two major parts: _The conscious mind_ and _the subconscious mind._

The Conscious Mind

The conscious mind is associated with wakeful thinking. It processes information from five major sensory points: sight, sound, touch, taste, and smell. As information comes in from these sensors, we can choose to retain it or ignore it. Because this processing is key, let us say that again: we can retain it or ignore it. The choice is ours.

In life we are constantly bombarded with things that are simply not true or many times, just not helpful in any way. Do any of these food-related "scoldings" sound familiar?

> "Clean your plate or you will not get dessert."
> "Eat all of your food! Don't you know there are starving children in Africa?"
> "I just spent all day cooking this food, so eat it."
> "Eat that food; it costs money and money does not grow on trees!"
> "Do not waste your food."
> "I do not care if you do not like it, eat it anyway."

And you are told that to lose weight you need to _____. *(fill in the blank)*

> eat less
> count calories
> reduce carbohydrates
> keep your heart rate above 120
> exercise at least two hours a day
> take these diet pills
> stop eating
> *(the list goes on and on, ad nauseam)*

The FYF4Good journey replaces these myths and mind games with the truth and teaches you what to do so you are always in control.

The Subconscious Mind

The subconscious mind can be thought of as the part of the mind that controls "feelings" (what we are seeing, hearing, touching, tasting, and smelling), as well as controls the body. Babies function with the subconscious mind. They are essentially sponges; they absorb everything. That is why they learn so fast. During the first year of life, a baby's brain will double in size, a tremendous, exponential growth. There are no filters telling the baby what is wrong or what is right. If we encourage babies and children with praise, their resulting confidence and success as an adult is astronomical. They learn languages quickly because they are using their subconscious mind. The conscious mind has not yet learned to filter what the baby hears, allowing all of the words and sentences to flow into their subconscious mind.

Once thoughts and ideas enter the subconscious mind, they do not leave *unless* new thoughts, a new way of thinking is consciously made. This can occur in one of two ways: (1) by a jarring event (usually these are bad things like an accident, trauma, or loss) or (2) by repetitive behavior. Regardless of which way it occurs, we can call this a "Paradigm Shift."

FYF4Good will take you through a huge Paradigm Shift, via repetitive behavior. This Paradigm Shift will challenge and reprogram everything you know, believe, and feel about food and the need to nutrify your body. Flush Your Fat 4Good: *Be Lean and Healthy for Life!* If you are twenty pounds or more overfat, out of shape, or just unhealthy, most likely you are trapped in a vicious cycle.

Think hard about this vicious cycle if this is your cycle **now:**

The Current Vicious Cycle

1) **Your Current Picture**: Overfat or overweight, unhealthy, no clue, not understanding what and how to eat and nutrify to be healthy. You are "guessing" what you should be eating or *worse*, you think that starving (fewer calories) will help you lose weight.

2) **This Picture Causes Thoughts**: These thoughts occur in the conscious mind: "I am fat." "I am unhealthy." "I do not like myself." "I look grotesque." "I feel like a fat slob." "My clothes look terrible on me." "I look so ugly." "I am so embarrassed of how I look."

3) **These Thoughts Cause Feelings:** These feelings occur in the subconscious mind. Negative feelings cause depression and the vibration of the body to slow down.

4) **Feelings Cause Actions**: These feelings cause your body to do more of the same: emotional eating, starvation, depression, poor choices. Nothing changes or worse you keep gaining weight. The same actions create the same result and the vicious cycle continues.

What if we "shift the paradigm" and try this another way?

GET READY TO SHIFT YOUR PARADIGM TO A NEW CYCLE

1) **Create a New Picture (using Thoughts)**: A picture of what you want. Talk as if it has already happened. "I am lean." "I am healthy." "I understand how to eat." "I know how to nutrify my body." "I am in total control."

2) **New Picture (Thoughts) Cause Feelings**: Imagine how this new you will make you feel. "Wow, I like the way I look!" "I feel in control." "I am excited to learn more." "I feel stronger than ever before." "I feel really good after eating healthier foods."

3) **New Feelings Cause Action**: Since the feelings are good feelings, the body will start vibrating at a much higher frequency. It feels energized. It likes this new picture. FYF4Good will step you through the actions you need to take to get there.

4) **New Actions Produce New Results**: And guess what? Rapid fat loss will ensure the shift, because you will experience and see the results. You are on the road to the new you!

It just starts with desire, which will lead to knowledge, and that will lead to understanding that will bring happiness. It happens by following the 8 Essential Pillars of the FYF4Good Lifestyle. Everything becomes a *Habitual Ritual!* The repetition of this Lifestyle causes the shift, a Paradigm Shift, to take place for a new and healthier you!

With FYF4Good you will never buy another diet book, join a weight loss center, take diet pills, consume diet smoothies, meal replacement shakes or bars, buy prepackaged fake food, start another "fad" diet, spend another dime on another gimmick, or spend an hour running on a treadmill to lose fat! Keep reading! You have what you need in your hands. Flush Your Fat 4Good is going to change your life, allowing you to eat yourself lean and never feel hungry or deprived again!!! You are in control now. Get ready to ROCK!

RESULTS TO EXPECT WHEN YOU FOLLOW THE FLUSH YOUR FAT 4GOOD LIFESTYLE

Whether you have twenty, or one hundred plus pounds of fat to lose, you are overfat! Your health is only going to get worse if you do not take action quickly. Do not wait one more day. If you follow the FYF4Good *Lifestyle to a "T"* the progress will be fast, it will be drastic, and the results will be life changing! What does following the FYF4Good *Lifestyle to a "T"* mean? It means you follow the rules exactly. Every minute of every day you do not deviate. You stay true to Phase 1 until *all* of the fat is burned off your body and then you move into Phase 2. Keep reading and you will learn why this is important.

What should one expect from FYF4Good?

- **Your body will return to having normal endocrine functions,** within a very short window of time. This is important because your endocrine system helps to regulate all of the major organs in your body.
- **Your production of insulin will be greatly reduced** and your body will begin to use the insulin produced more efficiently (seventy-two hours for most).
- **Water will be excreted rather than excessively stored.** The scale will register a dramatic weight loss (similar to other programs) within the first few weeks, mainly from water weight. But then something very exciting happens. Your body begins to shrink because you are **burning fat.** Within one to four weeks, or ten to fourteen days for most people, of following the FYF4Good *Lifestyle to a "T"* the body will go into Nutritional Ketosis, a state of safe, rapid fat loss. Fat deposits are used for energy. Fat is High Octane Premium Fuel. Burning fat for fuel is what the body was designed to do.
- **You may experience a D.O.E. (Day of Exhaustion).** This is a time to celebrate! This is the day when your body makes the switch to burn your own stored fat for fuel, rather than the foods

you are eating. You may experience the need to "crash on the couch" and not want to get up. Do not worry, it will not last long, a day or two at the most. If you have a lot to lose, you may experience this more than once. Even though you feel exhausted, it is a great thing! Feel excited about it! Listen to your body and rest when you need to.

- **After your D.O.E. you enter the Accelerated Fat Burning State**, or Nutritional Ketosis (Keto-Adaptation). You want to stay in this state until you reach your goal. This will happen if you follow the FYF4Good *Lifestyle to a "T"*!
- **Your body will start to look shapelier and firmer** as you develop lean muscles and burn the stored excess fat around your muscles.
- **Bone density**, **as well as overall health,** increases for most people.
- **Swelling and inflammation in the joints is reduced.**
- **Women should expect to lose ten to twelve pounds of FAT per month. Men should expect to lose twelve to fifteen pounds of FAT per month.** Why do men lose fat faster than women? Males make a lot of testosterone. Testosterone increases muscle mass. Muscle burns fat and increases metabolism. Fat is a stored energy source. Since males have more muscle mass, they burn the fat off more quickly.
- **Your visceral fat will decrease.** Excess visceral fat is very dangerous and cannot be removed with liposuction surgery. It is known as a "deep" fat that is stored further underneath the skin than "subcutaneous" belly fat. It is a form of gel-like fat that wraps around major organs, including the liver, pancreas, and kidneys.
- **The likelihood of hip or knee replacement is reduced**. As the body becomes lighter, stress is taken off the joints and joint space will increase. Synovial fluid bathes and nourishes the joints. As the fluid moves more freely and there is less weight bearing down on the joint, the body will start to re-absorb the arthritic changes in the joint. Before and after x-rays show this to be true.

- **No more cravings**, including sugar and starches!
- **Your digestive system will return to normal function**. If you once thought pooping every other day was normal, you will be amazed when your digestive system starts to function as it was designed. Two to four bowel movements per day is normal in the FYF4Good Lifestyle.
- **Your sleep will greatly improve**. You will sleep more deeply and awake refreshed.
- **Many people come out of a brain fog** after losing a significant amount of fat on this Lifestyle. This brain fog is often due to an overgrowth of yeast in the body. As you come off sugar and starches, excess yeast will "die-off." This will further promote healing.
- **Because you will be carrying less weight on your body, you will have more energy.**
- **It is likely you will no longer need a nap**. Many people, who previously felt the very common afternoon drop in energy, now have more energy.
- **You will have less foot pain or problems with your feet** due to less weight pressing down on them.
- **Many people experience better lab values** in their blood work and other medical tests.
- **Many people ultimately are able to reduce their prescribed medications** (FYF4Good suggests consulting and working closely with your health care practitioner, teaming up to get the best results).
- **Your weight will cease to yo-yo up and down.**
- **Your mood and self-esteem are likely to improve and regulate.**
- **Your hormones will balance out.**
- **You will likely become both a happier and nicer person!** Cool, huh? ☺

Do not waste another day! Let's get started!

The 13 FYF4Good Rules

Without rules, how would you know if you are playing the game right? How would you know if you are on track to win? Without knowing the fundamental rules, the game is over before it ever starts. Knowledge is power. So let's get the basic FYF4Good rules on the table.

Rule 1: Follow the *Lifestyle to a "T"*

This means you must follow all of the rules and all 8 Essential Pillars of this Lifestyle. You cannot pick and choose, you must go all in. Follow these rules to create what we call, a "Habitual Ritual." You do not think about brushing your teeth twice a day, do you? Nor should you think twice about how you feed yourself to survive in the healthiest way. It becomes second nature to you.

There is a method to the FYF4Good madness! If you alter the rules or decide to skip something, you will *not* get the optimal and rapid results. Period! Those that choose to not follow this *Lifestyle to a "T"* because they alter this for their own comfort and do not give themselves enough time to benefit from FYF4Good, do themselves a huge disservice and will not get the optimal results. Read the Pillars and understand them. If you do not completely understand, ask. FYF-4Good is not hard, but for most people it will be new and somewhat foreign. It takes time to learn a new lifestyle, and this one is lifelong: *Be Lean and Healthy for Life!*

Here is an example. Sugars, flour, starch, and cow dairy products are removed in Phase 1 (see chapter three "Phase 1: Eating and Nutrifying to Lose the Fat"). Just as a pinch of sugar in the gas tank of a car may destroy the engine ... right? Just a pinch or bite of sugar, even artificial sugar, flour, starch, or cow dairy products can stop your progress and set the fat burning process back days to weeks and might actually cause you to gain weight! It is not worth it. This means if you are not supposed to eat something (sugar, flour, cow dairy products), it is not okay to eat "just a little." *When in Doubt, Lay Out!* If you are not sure if something is Phase 1 compliant, do not eat it. Do not take a chance. Stay the course, and you will see the results.

Rule 2: GET a BUDDY and/or a COACH

In order to maximize success, FYF4Good strongly recommends that you get yourself a Buddy (see "Pillar #8: Support & Accountability" in chapter two to learn about Buddies). It is great if your Buddy is someone you know: a friend, spouse, significant other, partner, relative, neighbor, acquaintance. But do not despair if you are not ready to share your journey with others close to you. You will have hundreds of Buddies available twenty-four hours a day in the Private Flush Your Fat 4Good "Buddies" Facebook Group to help and support you. Just reach out and connect. Most importantly, it is so much fun!

It is most beneficial to be open and honest with your personal Buddy and Coach. Do not worry or get hung up on mistakes. There is a learning curve, and we are all human. You are in control. Jump back in and do the next meal correctly. Connect with your Buddy (phone, text, Facebook or in person) daily, or a couple of times a day, if necessary, when you are first getting started until you feel confident. Ask questions or private message Buddies in the Facebook Group. Live troubleshooting is available on weekly support calls to help you succeed. Find strength in numbers! Support is everything when going through a Paradigm Shift.

Rule 3: When You Are Hungry, Eat!

Your body needs nutrients to survive, so eat. There is no measuring food or calorie counting with this Lifestyle. *Do Not OverEat! Do Not Under-Eat!* Some days you will need more food than other days. That is okay. The exciting thing is your body and brain will start telling you. FYF4Good *Trains Your Brain!*

Rule 4: No Cow Dairy Products

I can already hear the "But—." NO BUTS! For most people, cow dairy is not healthy. What you learned as a child was not correct. The fact that a cow has a different ratio of hormones in their breast milk than humans AND this milk grows a calf into a one-ton animal with three stomachs, should be your first red flag! Humans are not designed to digest the proteins in the cow's milk and as a consequence, cow dairy is mucus-forming and contains unwanted elements. "What about the calcium?" Calcium in cow's milk cannot be digested well, if at all. Drinking too much cow's milk causes bonding with iron and can make children iron deficient. The largest cow milk-drinking nations in the world have the highest rate of osteoporosis. You will not prevent osteoporosis by drinking calcium. You need protein and minerals to protect your bones.

Rule 5: No Sugar, No Artificial Sweeteners, No Artificial Coloring or Dyes

- Sugar is like cocaine on the brain. Studies show that eating table sugar has the same addictive effect on the brain as cocaine.
- Sugar stops digestion immediately. Eating protein and then immediately eating a sugary dessert will stop digestion.
- Sugar causes an insulin response and mood swings.
- Sugar causes a fatty liver.
- Sugar makes fat.
- Sugar is addictive.
- Cancer lives in and on sugar.
- One week eating large quantities of sugar will destroy brain cells.
- Sugar grows yeast in a petri dish as well as in the body. A high percentage of diabetics and overfat people are battling with yeast infections. Most people do not know they have yeast infections because the body gets used to it and the person thinks it is a normal part of life. Yeast can wreak havoc on your body, in your brain and in your life.
- Sugar lowers your immune system, encourages inflammation and will also contribute to lower back pain.
- Sugar dehydrates you.
- Processed sugar is not the same as sugars that naturally occur in fruits. So do not justify your consumption of table sugar by citing that the cranberry juice we use for CranFlush[*] has some sugar in it. Keep reading to learn about the benefits of CranFlush and how

---

[*] In chapter one, "Preparing for Day One of the FYF4Good Lifestyle," you will learn how to make CranFlush.

to make it. If the cranberry juice is unsweetened, the sugar on the label is the sugar that naturally comes in the cranberries. It is NOT the same thing as table sugar.

- Artificial sweeteners trigger the brain. The brain is alerted by the taste buds detecting the sweet taste, that you are eating sugar, which stimulates the sugar addiction. Diet drinks not only are a huge waste of money, they contain no nutritional value. In fact, studies show that drinking sodas (diet and regular) increase the likelihood that you will develop osteoporosis, or worse, can create harmful health conditions long-term and put fat on you! Saccharin has no food energy and no nutritional value. Saccharin is linked to several forms of cancer. Read the label. If you see high-fructose corn syrup, corn syrup or glucose syrup put it back on the shelf.

- And artificial colors are poison, poison, poison! They were designed to make a food more appealing to the eye, but there is absolutely no reason to put these in your body.

Rule 6: No Partially Hydrogenated Oils

The body cannot properly digest partially hydrogenated oils. These are oils that have been chemically altered and "hardened." Your first clue should be that in the hot weather, margarine does not melt. The process of making hydrogenated oils alone should tell you to stay away from it. The controversy is the level of **trans fat** and how it is processed. Trans fats are a man-made fat, formed when hydrogen is added to vegetable oils, making the oil more solid and less likely to spoil (the more solid the margarine, the more trans fat it contains). Trans fats have been shown to increase the "bad" cholesterol (LDL) in the body similarly to saturated fats, and they tend to lower the "healthy" cholesterol (HDL) when eaten in large amounts. Furthermore, trans fats may make blood platelets stickier. There is no set of standards for trans fats however; one tablespoon of margarine packs a whopping three grams of trans fat and two grams saturated fat.

Instead, use and enjoy quality cold pressed organic olive oils, coconut oils, avocado oils, and real butter preferably organic from grass fed cows. Some oils also come in spray forms to use when cooking. Read your labels. If you see "partially hydrogenated oil" on the label, put it down or if already in your pantry, throw it out!

Rule 7: No Synthetic Supplements

Synthetic supplements contain: coal tar, petroleum, petroleum by-products, ground-up rocks, iron shavings and/or chemicals. They are made in a lab, through science, and are a cheap way to make the supplements. However, our bodies are not designed to digest ground up rocks or by-products of the oil refining process.

This Lifestyle, when followed **to a "T"** is designed to help you remove toxins and excess fat from your body. Do not put more toxins in by taking synthetic supplements.

Do not fool yourself by thinking that if the label says "supplement" or "vitamin" or "good for you" or "natural" that it is healthy. A great example of this is beta carotene. In the mid-1800s, scientists discovered how to extract, isolate, and synthesize beta carotene from the vitamin A complex. Vitamin A was the first fat-soluble vitamin discovered and includes other compounds such as retinol, retinal, retinoids, carotenes, and carotenoids in the whole complex. Beta carotene is only one piece of the whole vitamin A complex.

In the US CARET study (randomized, double-blind, placebo-controlled trial), more than eighteen thousand male and female asbestos workers and smokers were given a 30 mg supplement of beta carotene or a placebo. Scientists were testing if beta carotene could prevent lung cancer. The study was halted twenty-one months early because subjects receiving the beta carotene showed a 28 percent increase in incidence of lung cancer, a 17 percent increase in incidence of death, and a higher rate of cardiovascular disease mortality as compared to the control group on a placebo.

Do you understand the significance of this? They were trying to prove that a daily combination of 30 mg of (synthetic) beta carotene and twenty-five thousand IU of retinyl palmitate would reduce the incidence of lung cancer in two groups known to have higher lung cancer rates. Instead, the study was halted early because lung cancer rates and mortality *increased!* It would have been better to have given them a plate of raw organic carrots to receive the whole complex of Vitamin A. And still, these synthetics are used in over 90 percent of nutritional supplements on the market!

It is beneficial for the body to receive the whole natural food complex so it can be recognized, processed, and utilized. Beta carotene is just one part of the vitamin A complex found in nature. Without the whole complex of vitamins or minerals, the body cannot recognize it and thus waits for the rest of the parts to come in from the diet to make a complete complex. If they do not come in, then the body will leach from the bones, blood or tissue, to make a complete complex vitamin or mineral for utilization. In other words, your body will cannibalize itself just to make a complete complex that it can recognize and use. Therefore, after a while of using synthetics, you become more deficient than before you started taking the supplements.

On FYF4Good only whole-food plant-based supplements are taken. One hundred percent (100 percent) of the ingredients come from plants that provide nutrients needed by the human body in its full complex form.

For more information about the specific supplements recommended for this Lifestyle, continue reading and visit FlushYourFat-4Good.com.

Rule 8: No Preservatives

Read the label. If it contains Sodium Nitrates, Sodium Nitrites, EDTA, Sodium Sulfite, BHA and BHT put it back on the shelf or throw it out. There is also a flavor enhancer called MSG (Monosodium Glutamate). These chemicals are added to extend the life of food, sometimes for years, are not fresh sources and are not beneficial for the human body. In many cases, the food industry designed these dead foods to help you to become addicted. (Read *The Cost of Being Sick* by Nicholas J. Webb, June 1, 2003, if you want more information about the dangers in our foods and health care.)

Rule 9: No Processed Foods

It is simple. *If God made it, EAT IT! If man made it, READ IT!* You must understand what is put into the food. The best place to shop for most of your food is the perimeter of the grocery store. Many processed foods are designed to become addicting. Do not be fooled. Make it a habit to only put foods into your body that build, repair and maintain the integrity of your bones, blood, tissue, muscles, and organs.

Rule 10: A Big YES to Coffee!

WHAT? Yes, you heard right! The research is clear. Coffee has health benefits. Coffee is mandatory on FYF4Good (unless your religious beliefs restrict you from drinking coffee). Why? Here are some of the reasons:

It is a diuretic. That means it will help you eliminate retained water from your body.

It helps to get the bowels moving.

It increases metabolism.

It has been shown to help reduce the risk of certain cancers, such as breast cancer and melanoma.

It is a mood elevator.

It is an antioxidant. Studies show that it has some of the best antioxidant properties in the modern Western diet!

It enhances the brain function. Sharpens your mind, makes you smarter!

One-quarter cup to three cups daily is beneficial for you.

Organic coffee is a must! Nonorganic coffee is one of the highest pesticide sprayed crops in the world! Dark roast is lower in caffeine as it has been roasted out of the bean. If your body is sensitive to caffeine, dark roast is the one for you. Medium roast has more of a kick due to the caffeine.

Studies show that coffee increases your life expectancy.

Rule 11: Don't Be Foolish!

Just because there is no calorie counting and no food measuring does not mean to go wild. For example, goat and sheep cheese are allowed on Phase 1. That does not mean you should eat a pound of goat cheese every day, especially the hard cheeses. Your body will let you know you have done too much. Listen carefully to your body. I guarantee you will not be stuffing yourself with goat cheese the next day. Eat cheese to enhance or add flavor to the food. Learn to make smart decisions for your health. Follow **"13 FYF4Good Rules"** in this chapter and **"The 8 Essential Pillars"** in chapter two, AND use good judgment. *You want this fat off like yesterday, right?*

Rule 12: Forgive Yourself If You Make a Mistake

We all have! We bought the sweetened soy milk instead of the Organic, Unsweetened, Plain, non-GMO Soy Milk and did not realize for two weeks. Bummer! We went out to dinner and forgot pasta was not allowed in Phase 1. Ouch! We thought that eating less was better and were frustrated that we were not losing fat faster.

Remember, our biggest learning moments, the ones that last with us forever, often come from mistakes. It is just a MIS...TAKE! So when you figure out what your mistake was, recognize it, and do another "take." You are breaking habits, many of which have been with you for almost your entire life! Enjoy and be grateful for the journey!

Rule 13: Have Fun!

This is the most important rule of all. Have faith in the process. In the beginning, especially if you have a lot of fat to lose, and you have not quite figured out how this all works, this might be the most difficult rule to follow. But I guarantee you, if you stick with it, you will be having fun before you know it. Why? Because you will have lost your addictive behavior to food, your body will be getting leaner and healthier, you will understand what your body is doing with the nutrients you are putting in it. You will absolutely know that your health is improving. But more importantly you will feel it! You will have more energy. Your clothes will be looser. Your joints will have less soreness. Your mind will be clearer. You will be able to go out to eat at any restaurant and know how to order. You will experience freedom because you have learned the rules of the game, the Game of Life!

You will enjoy food for the first time in your life because you will be able to taste it, not have any guilt, eat until you are satisfied and are no longer hungry! Your relationship with food will be one of joy. You will have a sense of real control and confidence like you have never had before. Telling the waiter you want grilled or steamed vegetables instead of fries or baked potato, you want the two sides for your meal both vegetable dishes, to leave off the breading on the chicken or do not bring the hot rolls. You are finally in control of your destiny because you know what to do, and it will feel so good!

The most amazing experience is when you are out with your friends and you practice this Lifestyle. They will see someone who really has respect for themselves and their body and is serious about longevity and health. They inevitably will say, "I have got to start doing what you are doing!" "Maybe I will feel better and start to lose fat like you!" AWESOME! You have just changed their life! Get them involved if they are ready, and pay it forward!

Never give up! Stick with it. It becomes really fun. You will see results all along the journey. But more important, you are changing your health for life!

CHAPTER ONE

PREPARING FOR DAY ONE OF THE

FYF4GOOD LIFESTYLE

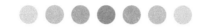

A Guide to Your First Twenty-Four to Forty-Eight Hours

Welcome to FYF4Good! Be INSPIRED, EXCITED, and HAVE NO FEAR about your first day! You will not regret your decision to take control of and improve your health and wellness! We know you want to get started as quickly as possible and not wait until you have finished reading this book. We do not blame you!

It takes time and practice (and mistakes!) to learn how this Lifestyle works. You must follow every piece of this *Lifestyle to a "T"* to lose your fat rapidly and safely. But there is much you can start doing right now, today. How many times have you told yourself, "Oh I will start my diet on Monday!" or "After the holidays!"? You will learn very quickly this is not a "diet"; it is *A Lifestyle for a Lifetime* and you need to jump right in! You can get started on your journey while you stock your pantry and refrigerator with the great foods you will need. Start the eating part before your supplements arrive. When they do arrive, you will have everything you need for fantastic success! It is ok to do this step by step until you have got it and own it. The faster you get the hang of it, the faster the results!

This chapter is designed to be a reference point to get you up and running quickly. It has information on what you can start doing immediately so that you will be ready to accelerate at high speed and have much success with this Lifestyle. But you must read the entire book to get all the information to insure optimal success. Some things will take some time, like figuring out which stores near you sell the items that you will need. Do not be discouraged with the learning process. Knowledge is power and educated people make educated decisions. So, as you are reading the book, we recommend a few steps to start following to prepare for what is to come.

JOIN OUR COMMUNITY OF AMAZING BUDDIES AND COACHES WITH A CULTURE OF CARING

To truly commit to this Paradigm Shift of *A Lifestyle for a Lifetime* we invite you to join our community. Go to FlushYourFat4Good.com and request access to the private Flush Your Fat 4Good "Buddies" Facebook Group. Watch, read, listen, engage, and learn. We have over one hundred Coaches ready to answer any questions you have. Learn from other Buddies that post their experiences. Get inspired by their changes and find some great recipes that Buddies are posting that are allowed for Phase 1 and Phase 2. One of the most important Pillars of FYF4Good is Pillar #8: Support & Accountability. We are all here for you to achieve your goal and to never, ever struggle again with fat loss.

PREPARE FOR SUCCESS

Before you start this journey, do yourself a favor and take a few minutes to remove everything from your pantry and refrigerator that might prove to be a stumbling block to your success. This would include all processed foods, such as cereals, chips, cookies, candy, ice cream, packaged meals, breads, pastas, and potatoes. You will not be eating these, so get rid of them!

SHOPPING GUIDE FOR THE GROCERY STORE

The next thing to do is a shopping trip to the grocery store. Always read the labels first. *If God made it, EAT IT! If man made it, READ IT!* So when buying the "legal" foods for Phase 1, keep this in mind: Buy organic foods if they are available and foods marked as cage-free, grass-fed, and antibiotic-free when possible. Never buy anything that has added nitrates, nitrites, EDTA, sugars, vinegar, synthetics, partially hydrogenated oils, dyes, or big words you cannot pronounce.

Here is a quick list of what you will need for Phase 1:

- Eggs
- Chicken (The whole chicken, chicken breasts, legs, or thigh meat are all good.)
- Turkey breast, turkey legs, turkey thighs (Turkey wings are also great.)
- Vegetables: Choose fresh low-glycemic, non-starchy vegetables.

    Here is a short list, but you can search online for non-starchy vegetables to see a larger list: broccoli, cucumber, onion, kale, arugula, bell pepper tomato, zucchini, cauliflower
- Lemons (You will need lots of these, so stock up.)
- Low-glycemic fruits

    Here are some ideas: apples, strawberries, red grapes, pears, blueberries, blackberries, kiwi, mango, cherries, peaches, nectarines, apricots, and papaya

    Note: No bananas or avocado on Phase 1
- Mayonnaise, organic (if available), unsweetened, non-GMO, EDTA-free (a preservative). You can also make homemade mayonnaise. Find this recipe and others in the Facebook Group or on FlushYourFat4Good.com.
- Dill Pickles *(no sugar, colors or chemicals, Trader Joe's brand is great)*
- Shallots (or other onions)
- Organic, unsweetened, plain, non-GMO Soy Milk *(Stock up on this!)* Goat, hemp, or flax milk can be substituted, but soy is preferred over hemp or flax because it is higher in protein.
- Organic Coffee (Buy organic dark or medium roast coffee. No flavored coffees!)
- Seasonings:

    Pink Himalayan Salt. You will use a lot of this, so buy a big jar *(find at Costco).*

    You can buy sea salt if you cannot locate the Pink Himalayan Salt.

    Montreal Steak Seasoning *(find at Costco)*

Organic No-Salt Seasoning *(find at Costco)*

cinnamon

pumpkin pie spice *(optional, find at Trader Joe's—available seasonally)*

cayenne pepper

- Cranberry Juice: This must be unsweetened, not from concentrate, 100 percent cranberry juice *(Be sure to stock up on this!)*
- Yogurt: This must be organic, unsweetened, plain goat or sheep yogurt *(or make your own)*
- Soy yogurt for vegans: This must be organic, unsweetened, plain soy yogurt *(or make your own)*
- Raw nuts or seeds; great choices are:
  walnuts, pecans, organic unpasteurized almonds, sunflower seeds, pumpkin seeds, macadamia nuts, hemp seeds *(no soaking required)*
- Three large glass bottles, Voss bottles are great, *(approximately twenty-seven ounces for a total of eight-one ounces a day)*.

ORDER YOUR SUPPLEMENTS

Keep reading the book to learn more about why we all must take supplements. A recommended supplement list is kept up to date and available on FlushYourFat4Good.com so you can easily find companies we recommend to buy them from.

PREPARE YOUR FOOD THE DAY BEFORE
Soak the Raw Nuts and Seeds

The reason raw nuts are soaked in salty water is because the salt acts to awaken enzymes that are then able to break down and neutralize enzyme inhibitors. Therefore, after soaking there may be evidence that your nuts or seeds have started sprouting. To soak them, put the raw nuts (a good amount to last you for about a week—about seven large handfuls!) in a bowl, leaving at least a two-inch clearance to the top of the bowl. Add about a tablespoon of Pink Himalayan Salt. Fill the bowl with filtered water so that the nuts or seeds are covered with water. Stir to mix the salt into the water. Cover the bowl with a lid and allow the nuts to soak at least seven hours. Overnight is best.

When soaking is complete, strain and completely rinse the nuts or seeds with fresh water. You will know when to stop rinsing as the water will be clear. After draining well, place paper towels on a cookie sheet and place the nuts or seeds onto the paper towels and spread out flat. Place in a warm oven (approximately 170 degrees Fahrenheit) for one to one-and-one-half hours. Stir and check to see if they are dry about every thirty minutes until drying is complete (nuts and seeds take different times to dry). Remove from oven, allow them to cool. Use a paper towel to pat dry if still a little moist. Place in a Ziplock bag or glass jar and store in the refrigerator. They will not be salty. The salt is rinsed away in the process.

From time to time for something different, after drying, spray the pumpkin seeds with an organic coconut or olive oil spray, sprinkle a little Pink Himalayan Salt (and cayenne pepper if a little extra flavor is desired) and return to the oven for more drying. The sprayed oil will allow the seasoning to stick.

Cook the Chicken

Rinse the skinless, boneless chicken breasts and pat dry. It is best to cook with a grill pan to give those great grill marks on your chicken. Put organic olive oil in the bottom of the grill pan to lightly cover the whole pan. Sprinkle Montreal Steak Seasoning and Costco No Salt Seasoning to lightly cover the pan. While the oil is heating, either cut your chicken breast into strips or filet it open to be flat. You want more area of the chicken breast to touch the pan. When the oil is hot, place the chicken in the hot oil laying it across the grill marks. Grill the chicken until it is golden brown.

After the chicken has cooled enough to handle, cut it up into small pieces. Make Jackie's Chicken Salad (detailed in chapter nine: "FYF-4GOOD Staples"). All of the ingredients are on the preceding shopping list.

DON'T FORGET TO PREPARE YOUR CRANFLUSH

With filtered water, fill a tall glass bottle (800 ml), 80 percent full. Fill to the top with unsweetened, not from concentrate, 100 percent cranberry juice. You may make it weaker by diluting a little if it is too strong at first. Prepare three of these bottles for the day. Take the recommended supplements with your CranFlush and with your fruit. To learn more about all of the FYF4Good recommended supplements read "Pillar #4: Nutrifying" in chapter two or visit FlushYourFat4Good.com. If you are still waiting for your supplements, drink the CranFlush without them until they arrive!

Get a Buddy and Make it Fun

If you do not have a Buddy, please go to the Flush Your Fat 4Good "Buddies" Facebook Group and post that you need a Buddy. Seriously think about asking a friend or family member to be your Buddy. Make it fun and find a partner! This creates accountability and support which in turn creates long-term success.

Day 1 – Get Off to a Good Start

First thing when your feet hit the floor in the morning it is time for breakfast. Go to the kitchen and "break your fast" by eating a large bowl of low-glycemic fruit (any or all apples, grapes, blueberries, strawberries, blackberries, nectarines, peaches, etc. You can mix them up. (Refer to "Selecting Fruits and Vegetables" in chapter eleven for other ideas.)

After you have swallowed the last bite of fruit, if you have received your recommended supplements, take the morning supplements with your CranFlush. Pour at least six ounces of CranFlush in a glass if it is easier for you to swallow your supplements that way.

You must wait twenty minutes after you eat your last bite of fruit before you have your FYF4Good Latte. Look at the clock and make a mental note or set the kitchen timer.

Use the twenty minutes to prepare your morning FYF4Good Latte. Make one to two cups of organic dark or medium roast coffee. Heat one (one-and-one-half if you prefer) cup of recommended milk. Recommended milk is NEVER cow dairy. See chapter nine: "FYF4GOOD Staples" for the recommended milks. Sprinkle cinnamon all over the top of the milk while heating. You may add a dash of cayenne pepper (it is a great thermogenic and tastes fantastic!)

Milk can be heated in a "frother," which will make it a fluffy treat. You can also buy a whisk and whisk the milk into froth. Pour coffee and milk into a sixteen to twenty-ounce mug. Add two scoops of your *FYF-4Good Super Lean Aminos (Muscle Building-Fat Burning Powder)*, making it approximately twenty grams of protein. Mix well and enjoy. It should take no more than thirty minutes to drink your FYF4Good Latte. Put in a travel mug and take with you if you are on your way out the door. To learn more about all of the FYF4Good recommended supplements see "Pillar #4: Nutrifying" in chapter two or visit FlushYourFat4Good.com.

EXERCISING

At least five days out of the week, at some point during the day, you will need to get a minimum of thirty minutes of walking. If possible, brisk walking without interruptions is best. However, go at a pace that you can handle in the beginning. If you cannot walk, do some sort of activity such as exercises while sitting. (Refer to "Pillar #7: Exercise & Sleep" in chapter two.) Put the time down on your schedule and make it happen!

After you have finished your FYF4Good Latte, eat your first protein meal within sixty minutes. FYF4Good *Trains Your Brain* to let you know what protein would satisfy you the most at this time. It could be Jackie's Chicken Salad, Jackie's Three-Egg Omelet, Jackie's Egg and Veggie Muffins, or goat yogurt with nuts.

One of the most common dishes for this first meal of the day is Jackie's Three-Egg Omelet with lots of low-glycemic vegetables and goat or sheep cheese (cheese is optional). Whisk the three eggs and pour into a lightly greased fry pan. Coconut oil, olive oil or organic butter from grass-fed animals works great. When the eggs are almost cooked like a pancake, turn it over and add your vegetables right down the middle. Chopped-up broccoli tops, tips of asparagus, mushrooms, zucchini, shallot, Bermuda onions, red bell peppers, a few leaves of kale or arugula, and perhaps some fresh salsa are all good. Then add a couple of soft dollops of plain goat cheese. Flip half of the egg pancake over the vegetables, grate a little sheep cheese (pecorino), over the top for a final touch and then put on a lid and turn down the heat. This allows your vegetables to slightly steam and the cheeses to soften. This dish should fill you up and keep you satisfied for about four hours.

If you make the omelet with six eggs, you can save one-half for later (steam it to reheat). You can do the same combo of a dozen eggs and vegetables and pour the mixture into a greased muffin tray. Place a dollop of goat cheese in the middle, a teaspoon of fresh salsa or Hatch Valley

Salsa from Trader Joe's, and grate a little pecorino sheep cheese on top. Bake for approximately twenty-two minutes at 350 degrees Fahrenheit or until they are golden brown. These egg muffins can be reheated by steaming or just take them in a Ziplock bag to snack on when room temperature.

For lunch or your next protein meal, have a bowl of Jackie's Chicken/Turkey/Tuna/Egg Salad on a bed of kale and arugula. This should also fill you up and keep you satisfied for about four hours. When you have swallowed your last bite of your protein meal, make note of the time. It takes four hours for protein to digest.

When four hours have passed, you will start all over again. Eat a large bowl of fruit, similar to the one you ate in the morning. Take your evening supplements. Look at the time and wait twenty minutes or set the timer if you need a little extra reminder. Fix another FYF4Good Latte. If you are affected by caffeine late in the day, try using the dark roast coffee. If it still affects you, leave the coffee out of this Latte, and just have the milk, cinnamon, two scoops of the *FYF4Good Super Lean Aminos* and cayenne pepper (optional). From one to three cups of coffee per day are allowed. Refer to the book's introduction listing "The 13 FYF4Good Rules" for the many health benefits of coffee. Enjoy!

About thirty to sixty minutes after your FYF4Good Latte, you will probably be hungry. Have some more Jackie's Chicken Salad, or perhaps goat yogurt with nuts, or grilled salmon with grilled asparagus. Maybe eat the second half of that egg omelet, whatever you feel like for a protein and vegetable meal. This should satisfy you for about four hours.

Many Buddies love goat yogurt with a handful of nuts before bed. Some Buddies, especially in the hot months, feel like having another bowl of fruit. Remember, FYF4Good *Trains Your Brain* to choose wisely! And always: *Do Not Overeat! Do Not Under-Eat!*

Did you get your thirty minutes of brisk walking (exercise) today? If no, it is not too late. Throw on those walking shoes and go walk around the block for the next thirty minutes. If it is too cold or unsafe, walk around your house for thirty minutes without stopping. Get on the Facebook Group or FlushYourFat4Good.com for ideas. There are also exercises there for those who cannot walk. Listen to music! Make it fun!

No excuses! You want to trigger the brain for fat loss so when you stop, you are still burning fat.

Just before bed, have your probiotic and then brush your teeth. Sweet dreams and plan to do day two just the same as day one.

A Very Important Routine to Follow

Check in with your Buddy and/or Coach every day, every other day—or whatever it takes— but at least once a week during the first month of your new Lifestyle. Get involved in the Facebook Group. This is an incredible supportive community, a culture of caring individuals and a great place to ask questions. Everyone in the group is cheering everyone on to reach their goal with no judgment. You will experience this the first moment you join and announce yourself. And please do introduce yourself once you are added to the Facebook Group. There is no negativity, no shame and only good will and support. Those that do not have support at home or from friends, you will find support here.

Get on the live support calls. This is a great place to ask questions and possibly have the creators, Jackie Padgette-Baird and Dr. Victoria Arcadi, troubleshoot you! This will help you to keep on track, never have doubt or question what you are doing, and see that you are part of an active, caring community. Being part of the support community is a vital part of the Lifestyle, as discussed in chapter two, "Pillar #8: Support & Accountability."

When you make a mistake (and we ALL do) do not get discouraged. Do not think that this Lifestyle is too hard. Do not think that you are the only person who will not succeed at this. These thoughts are natural, but they are *not true!* Call/text/email your Buddy or Coach. Go into the Facebook Group and private message any Buddy or post your questions. Get the information that you need and commit to start fresh and to do this Lifestyle correctly. Start with the next thing that you put in your mouth. *Do not be hard on yourself.* There is a learning curve in the beginning. Stay in the present, do not beat yourself up for the past or give an excuse to wait until tomorrow, focus on now. If you stay with it long enough, your Lifestyle will be one of clean eating, healthy habits and leanness.

Remember—You Can Never Go Wrong Eating Right!

CHAPTER TWO

INTRODUCING THE

8 ESSENTIAL PILLARS

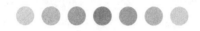

Flush Your Fat 4Good to Be Lean and Healthy for Life

Pillar #1: Nutritional Ketosis

Your body achieves this state when your brain turns on your body to burn your own stored fat for fuel, instead of your food. This Pillar is *key* to rapid, safe fat loss and the success people are experiencing with FYF4Good. The following seven Pillars are the secrets to success with Pillar #1 and all Pillars combined produces the results!

Pillar #2: Food Combining

It is all about digestion, absorption and elimination. This takes the burden off the digestive system by properly combining foods for maximum absorption of the nutrients in the food. Proper food combining means that certain food groups are not eaten together. This is basic physiology, allowing time for the stomach to empty between food groups. If food combining is not followed, foods could potentially putrefy (rot) in the gut. You will know this is happening because there will be symptoms such as burping, gas, heartburn, fatigue, lack of energy, bloating, stomach discomfort and constipation. Optimal digestion, absorption and elimination will be impaired, and the effect can include fat gain.

Pillar #3: Low-Glycemic Eating

This Pillar helps your body to maintain consistent blood sugar levels without instigating an insulin response. If low-glycemic eating is not followed, there will be spiking and crashing of blood sugars, which may lead to insulin resistance, whereby fat will be stored instead of burned. We are trying to get rid of fat, not store more of it!

Pillar #4: Nutrifying

Supplementing with whole-food nutrients to aid the body in its support and function, especially during rapid fat loss, is vital. In 1949 the United States Government announced that due to modern farming practices, our food no longer provides all of the necessary nutrients our bodies need for optimal health. The recommendation was to supplement. It is now prudent to take nutritional supplements for good health. It is well known that during any weight loss program, supplementation is recommended to help support the body and the cellular functions. This is a very important step that will encourage safe rapid fat loss, detoxing, flushing, cell repair and rejuvenation.

Pillar #5: Detoxing

Our bodies are exposed to toxins every day from the air, water, pesticides, preservatives and additives in our foods. Many of these toxins become stored in the body. Toxins are stored in your tissues, but mostly inside the fat cells. As you burn fat you will be releasing and eliminating these toxins. It is essential to protect your body from the toxins as they are eliminated. This is why Pillar #4: Nutrifying is extremely important. As the fat cells break up, antioxidants will help protect the cells from the toxins being released. Detoxing a lifetime of toxins in your body could be the healthiest thing you ever do but getting toxins safely out of the body leads us also to the next Pillar.

Pillar #6: Flushing

This Pillar is *key* to rapid fat loss and why we drink so much CranFlush. As fat is burned for fuel, it is circulating through the blood stream. Occasionally, it accumulates in the liver. Quickly flushing the fat and toxins out of the liver is very important. A clean and healthy digestive system and urinary system is vital for good health. This Pillar is designed to get these systems working in tip-top shape again. **FYF4Good is all interrelated and each Pillar supports the others.** The way we eat, the supplements we take, and the CranFlush we drink will each help you to have success with this Pillar.

Pillar #7: Exercise & Sleep

Thirty minutes of walking, five days a week, at a minimum, has been shown to be the ideal exercise to burn fat! If walking is not possible, do what you can to start moving. Activity in some form is the key. Additionally, sleeping is just as important for your health and success on FYF4Good. At least seven hours a night of continuous, restful sleep will insure optimal success! Read more about this Pillar to get ideas on how to accomplish both.

Pillar #8: Support & Accountability

Getting a Buddy, such as your spouse, sister, brother, friend, or neighbor to do this with you is a great way to get this Pillar started. Every week there are live support and trouble-shooting calls with certified FYF4Good Coaches and the creators, Jackie Padgette-Baird and Dr. Victoria Arcadi. This includes the Power100 Heroes Call, for people with a lot of fat to lose. For current schedules, details and more information, visit FlushYour-Fat4Good.com. In addition to the FlushYourFat4Good.com website, there is a Private (24/7/365) Flush Your Fat 4Good "Buddies" Facebook Group, Archived Calls, Coaches and Buddies—and more—you are not alone! Make this your Hub of Knowledge on how to be lean and healthy 4Good. You have never experienced anything like this and we look forward to welcoming you into the FYF4Good community, where you will find an incredible *Culture of Caring*.

PILLAR #1

NUTRITIONAL KETOSIS

An accelerated fat-burning state

Nutritional Ketosis (also called Keto Adaptation) is when your body is in an "Accelerated Fat-Burning State." If you apply Pillars #2 through #7 of FYF4Good: Food Combining, Low-Glycemic Eating, Nutrifying, Detoxing, Flushing, and Exercise & Sleep, your body will start burning the fat—and it will burn it fast, in a safe and healthy way. When this occurs, your body is in Nutritional Ketosis.

The main source of energy for the body is called glucose. Glucose is a form of sugar. *But wait a minute. One of the rules of FYF4Good is that we do not want to eat sugar, and now you are telling me sugar is needed to fuel the body?* Not all sugars are the same. In chapter eleven, the section "All Sugars Are Not the Same" will explain how sugars differ and what they do to our body.

Glucose is generated from breaking down the foods we eat and is stored as fat via a series of metabolic processes that occur in conditions when carbohydrates are depleted. Insulin in our body is used to turn glucose into glycogen. Glycogen is how we store glucose until we need to use it. Glycogen is needed for survival, but our bodies are able to only store about twenty-four hours of glucose.

What happens in the body when all of the glycogen is used up?

When our body is not taking in enough carbohydrates to supply the body with glucose (sugar), and all of the glycogen reserves have been used, fat is broken down. This occurs overnight when we are asleep, or when fasting or on a diet where food intake is restricted. Insulin levels are low during this time, but glucagon and epinephrine are normal. This combination signals the body to release fat from the fat cells into the bloodstream; it is carried to the liver where ketones (and ketoacids) are produced. The ketones (and ketoacids) travel from the liver, through our bloodstream, back out into the body where they are needed for energy (muscles, brain, and tissue).

Putting the body into Nutritional Ketosis means your body is in an optimal state to burn your own fat for fuel. Insulin is secreted at very low levels, consistently without spikes, which allow the adipocytes (fat cells) to secrete and release the fatty acids. Because your body needs are being met, the body will start burning fat! This is all done under the direction of the brain. And as you stay in this state, the fat will burn fast without jeopardizing muscle or bone. As a result, your energy and well-being will sky-rocket!

Did you know the Inuit tribes (one of which is commonly referred to as the Eskimos) have a diet that has maintained them in Nutritional Ketosis for more than three thousand years? The Inuit people live far to the north in Alaska, Canada, Siberia, and Greenland. They are totally influenced by the cold tundra climate and there are no grains or starches available for them to eat. This shows there is no issue about the "safety" of extended Nutritional Ketosis. It is very safe and provides rapid burning of stored fat for energy, which is the optimal fuel for the body.

Note: Nutritional Ketosis should never be confused with diabetic ketosis (ketoacidosis).

Please refer to the section "The Difference Between Diabetic Ketosis and Nutritional Ketosis" in chapter eleven to understand the difference.

PILLAR #2

FOOD COMBINING

Don't knock it until you try it!

Food combining is not difficult to learn or practice. It is just different than what most of us are accustomed to doing. Food combining is based on human physiology and it is not new. Two well-known nutritionists in the earlier part of the 20th century, Dr. William Howard Hay (1866-1940) and Dr. Herbert Shelton (1888-1987), promoted food combining. Dr. Shelton introduced food combining in his book published in 1951, "Food Combining Made Easy". Despite the title, it was still a very complex book. Dr. Hay's contribution, defining food combining, is considered so important that food combining rules are often referred to as the Hay Diet, and following them is known as "Haying". However, the general idea of food combining goes back to at least the 1850's when natural hygienists discovered that eating incompatible foods in the same meal could affect the digestion and absorption of valuable nutrients. With no disrespect to all the highly credible preliminary work carried out by Hay and Shelton, it would be wrong not to also give credit to Jan Dries, a renowned nutritionist from the Netherlands, who presented a completely new view of food combining in the 1970's. Those that still cannot accept the theory of food combining tend to assume that all foods contain basically the same nutrients and that simultaneously these nutrients are subject to the digestive process. In other words, they think all foods go down the same way and end up in the same place, so food combining is pointless.

For those truly seeking the most optimal health possible, food combining comes to their attention during their quest. Once you understand the simplicity of how your digestive tract works, food combining will not only make perfect sense, but instead of the fear of change, many feel it gives them hope. Why? Because once you try it, you see that it works! We have designed FYF4Good to be simple, easy and fun for lifestyle living. It is easy to be compliant with the FYF4Good food combining rules and the results are changing people's health for the better. People are amazed at how quickly digestive issues improve and fat loss occurs.

To understand the rules of food combining, you must first understand the basics of how the digestive system works. Digestion is KEY! The sole purpose of our digestive system is to break down the food we eat into the nutrients, or building blocks, needed to build, repair, and maintain the integrity of our bones, blood, tissue, muscles, and organs. Since 70 to 80 percent of our immune system is in the gut, it stands to reason that we need to have our digestive system functioning optimally. Please refer to the section in chapter eleven, "The Digestive System," for more details on how the digestive system works.

When digestion operates at peak performance, it occurs in a predictable daily cycle:

4:00 a.m. to Noon, ELIMINATION takes place
When we get up in the morning we "break the fast," BREAK-FAST. Our body has gone for eight to twelve hours without eating. It has burned through the glycogen reserves and if we are in Nutritional Ketosis, our body has been breaking down our fat to be used for fuel. Additionally, our body has now produced waste that needs to be eliminated.

When living the FYF4Good Lifestyle we start each morning with low-glycemic fruit, drink our CranFlush and take our supplements, our FYF4Good Latte, followed by the first protein meal of the day. This signals the body to start the process of elimination.

Noon to 8:00 p.m. is the time of APPROPRIATION
During this phase we are eating, the food is moving through the first stages of digestion to break the food down into nutrients the body can use. This occurs in the mouth, stomach, and small intestines.

8:00 to 4:00 a.m. is the time of ASSIMILATION

While we sleep, our bodies are busy with many important functions occurring primarily on the cellular level. Once the digested food moves into the intestines, these nutrient molecules are absorbed into the bloodstream and are sent to where they are needed. Assimilation is the movement of digested food particles into the cells of the body for use anywhere in the body. This is why sleep is so very important. During the time we sleep, the digested amino acids are forming proteins; and glucose is used in the cells for energy in the body. Healing, repair and cleansing, takes place in the cells. If we have healthy cells, we have optimal health. If our cells cannot get the proper molecular nutrients, we will not have optimal health. The human body is an amazing machine. If digestion is efficient and effective, the cells will get the nutrients they need.

Why Should We Combine Foods Properly When We Eat?

Food combining is done to achieve optimal digestion, absorption and elimination of the food we eat. It takes a tremendous amount of energy for our body to digest food. You want your body to devote the least amount of energy to digesting your food. Why? It has too many other things to do. Proper food combining makes it easy for the body to digest, fully absorb and eliminate the waste.

Think back to your chemistry class in high school or college. When you mix acid and alkaline together in a science beaker, what happens? They neutralize each other and become ineffective. The same thing happens in our stomachs.

In the human body, acid breaks down protein, alkaline breaks down starches. If you put protein (e.g. meat) and starches (e.g. potatoes) into your body at the same time, the digestive enzymes will not work because they become neutralized when they are combined in the stomach. As such, if food combining rules are not followed, the food can take double the time to digest, and will often putrefy (rot) in the stomach. Putrefaction becomes toxic, creates gas, bloating and discomfort when heat, acid and enzymes are applied to the mis-combined foods in your gut. The food stays in your stomach longer because it is not digesting well.

Once the putrefied food arrives in the intestinal tract, the probiotics are not able to utilize all the nutrition. The job of the probiotics is to extract nutrients and to send them throughout the body to build, repair and maintain the integrity of your bones, blood, tissue, muscles, and organs. This cannot happen effectively if the food is putrefied.

Think about when you eat a huge meal, maybe on Thanksgiving or another holiday. You often want to go lie down and rest after eating, don't you? The digestion process is exhausting on the body when we ask it to work harder than it is designed to work. Properly combining foods allows the acid enzymes (needed to breakdown protein) to work separately from alkaline enzymes (needed to breakdown starch). This is basic chemistry 101.

Digestive Enzymes

The three major types of digestive enzymes are:

- Amylases – these break down carbohydrates (starches, fruit) into glucose.
- Proteases – these break down proteins (found in meats, nuts, cheese, and yogurt) into amino acids.
- Lipases – these break down fat into its component parts.

If you eat food that requires amylases (high pH) with food that requires proteases (low pH), there will be stagnation in digestion and the digestive time will lengthen. It may take about eight hours for the food to adequately digest and empty out of the stomach. Your body may experience uncomfortable digestive symptoms and issues, and you can ultimately gain fat. You will not feel good. End of story! We see and hear about it every day.

"But I grew up eating meat and potatoes together!"

Take a clue from TV: Think about all the commercials we see on television for digestive problems: excess gas, acid reflux, constipation, and diarrhea. Products focused to "put band-aides" on the human digestive system are a multibillion-dollar industry. These products are designed to address the symptoms, not the problems. Most digestion problems are a result of mis-combining foods. If you follow the simple rules outlined here in FYF4Good, these issues will be reduced and very well may go away completely!

How We Made Our Choices for Food Combining

Food combining is based on human physiology. In 1951 Dr. Herbert Shelton wrote a book called *Food Combining Made Easy*. Every doctor studies human physiology and what is involved in digesting different foods, along with the enzymes necessary for digestion. But very few have utilized and applied food combining in their practices.

Nutrients are needed for every function in the body. Because we get our nutrients from what we eat, digestion is top priority in the body. Digestion is one of the hardest functions in the body. Proper food combining takes the burden off digestion.

Food combining as defined in Dr. Shelton's book is complicated and at times difficult to understand. The rules followed in FYF4Good have been simplified but are in compliance with Dr. Shelton's research. Why did we simplify them for FYF4Good? The goal is to obtain a *healthy Lifestyle for a Lifetime!* Whether you are a beginner or the more experienced, you should be able to do this in your sleep. We have simplified it for compliance reasons, so that anyone can food combine and get amazing fat loss results and better digestion, absorption and elimination. Later, if you so choose, you have the option to go even deeper into the food combining complexities for optimal health and well-being.

Herbert M. Shelton in *The Hygienic System, Vol II,* reports the works of Arthur Cason MD, who in 1945 conducted numerous experiments testing the efficiency of digestion throughout the digestive system when eating flesh (protein) with starches (carbohydrates) at the same meal. Dr. Cason found that after measuring the digestive rates, digestion is retarded and, in some cases, prevented. He went on to examine the fecal matter after it went through the entire digestive tract. He concluded that "Such tests always reveal that the digestion of proteins when mixed with starches is retarded in the stomach, the degree varying in different individuals, and also in the particular protein and starch ingested. An examination of the fecal matter reveals both undigested starch granules and protein shred and fibers, whereas, when ingested separately, each goes to a conclusion."

When food is combined properly, it is fully broken down, digested, absorbed, utilized by the body, and eliminated. Elimination would NOT include undigested fragments in the fecal matter. Incompatible combinations of foods cause fermentation, alcohol production in the digestive tract. It is quite possible that this alcohol production could potentially cause damage to the liver similar to drinking alcohol. It is very interesting to note here that today we now know that the most common liver disease in the United States is known as NAFLD (Nonalcoholic Fatty Liver Disease) where fat infiltrates the liver. It is also called "simple fatty liver." At the time of writing this book, it is estimated that 30 to 40 percent of the adults in the United States and 24 percent of adults globally have NAFLD. The incidence in the obese is 30 to 90 percent and in the obesity related conditions such as type 2 diabetes, the incidence is 40 to 80 percent. Approximately 20 percent of these people will have the hepatitis form called NASH (nonalcoholic steatohepatitis) where there is liver cell damage that may lead to cirrhosis and liver cancer, as well as fat infiltration in the liver.

Rules for Food Combining in FYF4Good Phase 1: Lose the Fat
Remember to Pay Attention to Your Food Groups

- **Fruit** can never be eaten at the same time as protein, starches or vegetables. *Always eat fruit alone on an empty stomach.* It only takes twenty minutes for your body to digest low-glycemic fruit. That is why in FYF4Good the first thing you eat in the morning is low-glycemic fruit to kick-start the digestive system. After eating fruit, wait at least twenty minutes before switching to your next food group.
- **Vegetable** carbohydrates will come from low-glycemic, non-starchy vegetables. Vegetables like broccoli, Brussels sprouts, asparagus, zucchini, kale, arugula, cauliflower, peppers, mushrooms, onions, etc. After eating vegetables, you must wait two hours before having fruit again, as fruit must always be by itself in the stomach. Vegetables should be hard to chew: raw, grilled or slightly steamed. If you are eating cruciferous vegetables (cabbage, broccoli, cauliflower, or Brussels sprouts) consider grilling or steaming. They

are fibrous and can be difficult to digest. Unless you are chopping the floret tops of broccoli into little bite sizes for Jackie's Chicken Salad, it is best to grill or very slightly steam your cruciferous vegetables before eating. See "Selecting Fruits and Vegetables" in chapter eleven for a partial list or use your internet search engine for "cruciferous vegetables."

- **Proteins** (meats, fowl, fish, goat/sheep/soy yogurt and cheeses, nuts, seeds) can be eaten at the same time as vegetables because the digestive enzymes do not neutralize each other. Additionally, when you eat protein, you must eat vegetables with it, as this helps push the food through. Eat hard to chew, crunchy vegetables with meat. Eat nuts/seeds with goat or sheep yogurt. You always want to be chewing your food. And *The Harder to Chew, The More You Lose!*

- **Do not mix "kinds" of protein**, for example land animal meat with fish (i.e. Surf and Turf), as they do not digest well together. If it walks, eat it with another protein that walks. If it swims, eat it with another protein that swims. If it is plant protein, do not mix it with animal protein. They each digest differently.

- **Proteins require four hours to digest** before you can eat fruit again. So, if you ate protein and vegetables, and two hours later you are hungry, eat more vegetables. This will allow you to only wait two more hours after the vegetables until your next fruit serving. However, if you are hungry for a protein, by all means eat more protein and vegetables. Listen to you brain. FYF4Good *Trains Your Brain* to tell you what your body needs, not what you want. Listen carefully and you will be amazed. It will tell you which food group you should be in at that moment of hunger.

Be aware that it takes your body one to four weeks of FYF4Good Phase 1 eating before your body goes into Nutritional Ketosis (Accelerated Fat Burning State). So, if you are on FYF4Good Phase 1, stick with it, do not mis-combine. Stay in the Accelerated Fat Burning State and get the fat off quickly. Eating a dessert or having a glass of wine will take you out of the Accelerated Fat Burning State for up to four weeks. You want this fat off like yesterday, right? So stay the course! (For more details see "Phase 1: Eating and Nutrifying to Lose the Fat" in chapter three.)

Rules for Food Combining in FYF4Good Phase 2: A Lifestyle for a Lifetime

- When you advance to FYF4Good Phase 2, you can eat both low and high-glycemic fruit (watermelon, pineapple, cantaloupe, banana). Just understand that high-glycemic fruit will take thirty minutes to digest, so you must wait a little longer before eating something other than fruit.
- You can add in starchy vegetables and grains: sprouted grains, Ezekiel bread, sweet potato, beans and rice, pasta, pumpkin, healthy roots.
- As in Phase 1, you must always keep in mind your food groups and do not mis-combine.
- Raw vegetables pretty much combine with everything, so you can consider them "neutral"—meaning they combine with any category (except fruit).
- Avocados are technically a fruit but also combine well with starches due to their fat and small plant protein fibers.
- Melons are best eaten alone.
- Sweet fruits are to be eaten alone.
- Do not eat acidic citrus fruits with other types of sweet fruits.
- When you eat a starch you always want to include a fat. This helps to keep the blood sugar from spiking. So, if you are having Ezekiel bread or sprouted ancient grains, spread on avocado, coconut oil, butter, raw organic nut butters, or olive oil. Only have one meal a day containing starch. You do not have to eat starch every day. If you let starches get out of control, go back to FYF4Good Phase 1 to regulate yourself. You will be back on track quickly. That is the beauty of Flush Your Fat 4Good. You are in total control!
- In FYF4Good Phase 2 if you want to eat sweets, eat the sweets on an empty stomach, choose carefully and really try to go healthy. Give your stomach a fighting chance and wait at least two hours

before eating something else. Sweets are a starch, which takes two hours to digest. Do this only on special occasions. Never have sweets two days in a row. Sugar is addictive and you do not want to go back into that addictive cycle.

- If you would really like to have a glass or two of alcohol, drink *before* eating: beer, tequila with lime and salt, or vodka. Dry red wine is also good. It has resveratrol which is linked to reducing the risk of coronary disease and cancer PLUS has anti-aging benefits. Do not add mixers that are sugary. Drink before your food arrives. Drinking on an empty stomach will mean that you will need less to feel the effects, and it will be easier on your digestive system. Do not pour alcohol onto food in your stomach. Drink and enjoy. Then eat.

- For best results, eat a starch meal after drinking alcohol. If that is not possible, eat the vegetables first and then eat the proteins. The purpose of this is to allow the alcohol to have time to exit the stomach before the protein is eaten.

- Drink alcohol in moderation. Excess alcohol messes up your kidney and liver functions. Many people have "fatty" livers and do not even know it. Do not be foolish.

You are working so hard for optimal health and leanness for a lifetime. Ask yourself how old do you want to be when you take your last breath? That might seem like an odd question but if you have an age in mind then you will think twice about what you put in your mouth. This is *Health by Design, Not by Default!* Live long and prosper. Why live long and suffer?! Whatever you do, treat your body for health and longevity in honor of the gift God has given you. For more details see chapter four, "Phase 2: Eating and Nutrifying."

DIGESTION TIMES OF FOOD GROUPS TO FOLLOW FOR FOOD COMBINING

FYF4Good uses very simple rules for combining food groups based on the length of time for foods to digest. Our goal is to make it as simple as possible to follow the food combining rules. This is so you will have greater success getting that fat off quickly and your digestive system functioning optimally as soon as possible. Here are the times it takes for digestion:

20 minutes	Low-Glycemic Fruit
30 Minutes	High-Glycemic Fruit
2 Hours	Low-Glycemic Vegetables (Non-Starchy)
2 Hours	High-Glycemic Vegetables (Starchy)**
4 Hours	Animal Proteins
4 Hours	Plant Proteins
2 Hours	Starch (Bread, Rice, Whole Sprouted Grains, Legumes, Potato, Beans, Cookies, Cakes, etc.)**

Exception
6 hours	PORK

** Phase 2 ONLY

PILLAR #3

LOW-GLYCEMIC EATING

Controlling the sugar levels in your bloodstream

Low-glycemic eating means fruits and vegetables are selected that will have minimal effect on glucose circulating in your blood. It also means no processed sugars and no flour. Even the sugar in a breath mint or chewing gum should not be consumed. The goal is to not instigate an insulin response in your body.

A food's glycemic index (GI) and glycemic load (GL) are the measurable effect on blood glucose after the food (containing carbohydrates) is consumed. Glycemic index is a measure of how quickly foods break down into sugar in the bloodstream. Glycemic load measures the amount of carbohydrates in a serving of food. On FYF4Good, we are only concerned with glycemic index. By eating low-glycemic fruits and vegetables (non-starchy) you will not instigate an insulin spike.

Low-glycemic fruits include: cherries, strawberries, blueberries, apples, red grapes, peaches, plums, mangoes, and papayas to name a few. Watery fruits are essential on Phase 1. Stick with fruits that have a GI below sixty. Also, always choose organic produce if possible, and try to get vine-ripened foods. Purchasing from a farmer's market is usually great as they often pick their fruit the day before. Vine-ripened fruit has the most phytochemicals for optimal cell protection, nutrients and taste.

There are a few exceptions. For example, bananas and avocados have a low-glycemic index but have no fluid in them. Save these fruits for Phase 2. They are healthy fruits, but they do slow down digestion. Most people do not need to have their digestion slowed down. *This is FLUSH Your Fat, not SLUSH Your Fat!*

In general, *The Harder to Chew, The More You Lose!* For example, cooked carrots have a high-glycemic index; raw carrots have a low-glycemic index. Examples of low-glycemic vegetables are broccoli, cucumber, cauliflower, zucchini, kale, arugula, peppers, mushrooms, asparagus, and Brussels sprouts to name a few. There are many choices. Refer to "Selecting Fruits and Vegetables" in chapter eleven for a list of common low-glycemic fruits and vegetables. You can also use your internet search engine to find more comprehensive lists of low-glycemic fruits and vegetables.

PILLAR #4

NUTRIFYING

There is no argument! Supplementing is essential!

Latest statistics indicate that a large majority of our population is micro-nutrient deficient and in need of proper supplementation due to poor food choices. So, before you say this chapter is not for you, read on! NOT ALL SUPPLEMENTS ARE ALIKE! In FYF4Good we only approve of whole-food sourced supplements. We are detoxing the body and do not want to put toxins, including synthetic supplements, which become toxic, back into the body.

The human body is not only a gift from God, but it is a very sophisticated machine. And like any top-notch machine, you need to take care of it. If you were driving a Lamborghini, would you put a low octane, cheap junk fuel in the gas tank? NO, of course not! The same should be true of your body. You only have one body in this life and you cannot trade it in every few years for a newer model. It needs high-grade, supreme octane, premium fuels!

What Are the Best Fuels for the Human Body?

First let's take a look at the worst—Synthetic Supplements! Did you know that over 90 percent of the supplements on the market are synthetically produced? That means they are made from coal tar, petroleum, petroleum by-products, ground-up rocks, iron shavings and/or chemicals. Our human bodies are not designed to recognize (let alone digest) these things. They quite often can be seen, undigested, on x-ray films or in the toilet.

Yuck! The human body cannot digest them because it is designed to only recognize and digest food!

Synthetic nutrition, developed in the 1930s, was born out of a need to produce dietary supplements to address vitamin-deficient conditions. After determining that supplementation was essential for certain health conditions (e.g. scurvy), scientists developed synthetic supplements (vitamin C). This new technology was used to try to replace what was deficient in the body by using chemical compounds developed in a lab. These chemical compounds are what we now know as pharmaceutical grade (USP) synthetic supplements.

Synthetic supplements are designed to have the same chemical properties as their naturally occurring counterparts, but they are not the same as nutrition found in nature. Chemists have had a very hard time trying to separate and isolate the many factors of vitamin C complex, for example. Vitamin C complex contains rutin, flavonoids, catechin, polyphenols, several enzymes and more. Vitamin C is much more than ascorbic acid, which is the synthetic form. Making supplements chemically is inexpensive, so they can be sold at a lower price. This makes them available to a larger segment of the population. However, they are no match for the benefits of taking the whole-food complex. In other words, synthetic vitamin C supplements do not work as well as eating limes and lemons. This was very evident when trying to treat scurvy with synthetic vitamin C or beriberi with synthetic vitamin B-1.

The production of supplements has evolved through time and now there is a second-generation of synthetic supplements that are coupled with food. This was an effort to supplement using real food with synthetics. The problem is these second-generation supplements are still made with synthetic chemicals from a lab. The synthetic nutrition in these food-based supplements are not recognized and digested well by the body.

A warning of caution when consuming synthetic substitutes: Some have been shown to have harmful effects on the body. The *New England Journal of Medicine* in 1995 and 1996 reported the results of studies on synthetic nutrition and its harmful effects. These studies showed that synthetic vitamins:

- Increased lung cancer rates by 46 percent
- Increased cardiovascular disease by 26 percent
- Increased mortality rates in forty-seven clinical trials
- Increased birth defects by 400 percent!

On FYF4Good, we do not recommend that *any* synthetic nutrition be consumed. Instead, real nutrition should be obtained from the foods we eat and from high-quality real whole-food technology supplements.

Natural whole-food vitamin and mineral supplements have high bioavailability, which means that more of it is recognized for immediate use by our bodies. Because only 5 to 7 percent of the nutrition of a synthetic vitamin and mineral is absorbed into the body, much more quantity is needed when taking a synthetic version. Why? The body cannot identify coal tar, petroleum, petroleum by-products, ground-up rocks, iron shavings and/or chemical vitamins and minerals. It does not matter if they are nanoparticles of rocks. A rock is a rock is a rock!!

Additionally, many synthetic supplements will become toxic to the body. They are not recognized as food; therefore they are stored or eliminated without any absorption or benefit. Prolonged use of mega doses of ascorbic acid, for example, has been shown to cause kidney stone formation and other vitamin deficiencies. Synthetic supplements have often been referred to by medical doctors as "expensive urine" because the nutrition is eliminated without being used.

Whole-food vitamin and mineral supplements are a little more expensive to extract and standardize and have a limited shelf life as compared to synthetic vitamin and mineral supplements, making them more expensive—but oh so much more beneficial! Pay now, or pay later!

The United States government announced in the late 1940s that our soils were depleted, our foods were deficient, and to achieve better health, the government recommended that its citizens take dietary supplements. In the past, many health care practitioners recommended that we did not need to supplement our eating with nutritional supplements. They knew the supplements were synthetic, and they had experience seeing the undissolved caplets captured on the radiographs in the colons of patients. Now, most health care practitioners recommend that we *do* need to supplement. The *Journal of the American Medical Association* reversed a long-standing anti-vitamin stance by publishing two scientific review articles recommending multivitamin supplements for all adults in 2002.

Why is there a shift in recommendation of supplements?

Due to our modern farming practices, which include green harvesting (picking fruits and vegetables before they are ripened), pesticides, herbicides, genetic modification (GMO), failure to practice crop rotation and resting of the ground (as outlined in the Bible and practiced for centuries), the vast majority of our foods are now extremely low in nutritional value.

This means that the right food supplements are necessary for maintaining good health.

Recommended Nutritional Supplements for FYF4 Good Lifestyle

1) **A whole-food multivitamin and mineral supplement** should be taken for good overall balance. We cannot live without vitamins and minerals. Vitamins play key roles in many biochemical reactions, which will not proceed in their absence, leading to sick cells and vitamin deficiency disorders. They are essential to the body for important functions. Healthy cells make healthy tissues, and healthy tissues make healthy organs. Healthy organs lead to healthy bodies.

   Minerals promote bone, hair, and skin health. They help the immune system to function. They play an important role in how energy is generated by the cells, and repair cell damage from chronic stress. Minerals are critical and aid in cellular processes and function of digestive enzymes, which translates to efficient basic body biological functions.

   The best choice of a multivitamin supplement is one that is whole-food. There are very few multivitamins out there made entirely from food. Multivitamins, found at the grocery store or drug store, are *not* going to cut it. To be healthy, you need a multivitamin and mineral supplement that comes from *all food*. We will help you find one.

2) A **glyconutrients (glycans) supplement** is highly recommended. Good cell-cell communication and cell-cell recognition is *mandatory* for your body's needs.

Scientists have discovered that cell-cell communication and cell-cell recognition occur on the surface of cells. The surface of every cell in your body is covered in hair-like structures called glycans which are chains of sugars that are linked to molecules such as specific proteins.

There are hundreds of different glycans on our cells, each with its own function. They are used for recognition, identification and communication. Many functions in the body, including how the sperm attaches to the egg, are dependent upon proper cell-cell communication and recognition. Immune cells, for example, will identify harmful viruses and bacteria and attach to them often via glycans. Then the immune cells will hopefully make sure that the invaders are destroyed. Our cells can also recognize hormones, again often via glycans and respond accordingly. Eight sugars make up many of the glycans found in humans. One of these is glucose, which of course is present in abundance in our diets. Some nutritionists claim that our modern day diet supplies only limited amounts of some of the seven other sugars.

Therefore, FYF4Good recommends a **glyconutrients supplement** to help our cells make our own glycans. Glyconutrients are often mixtures of plant glycans containing most of the eight sugars. These glycans must be broken down by enzymes in our digestive system and their individual sugars are then absorbed and used by our cells to build up human glycans.

3) **Antioxidants are important** to protect our cells from free radical damage and help eliminate toxins formed by free radical damage in our cells. Free radicals are connected to human disease, including cancers, atherosclerosis, Alzheimer's, Parkinson's and many oth-

ers. Free radicals can be found in the medicines we take, foods we eat, the air we breathe and the water we drink. They damage and cause oxidation or "rusting" of our cells linking them to premature aging. Toxins harbor in the fat cells, and when the fat cells start to break up and be eliminated, it is invaluable to have your other cells protected from free radicals with an effective antioxidant.

Every day our bodies are bombarded with toxins in our polluted environment. We are hit thousands of times a day by these toxins but do not realize it. Toxins should be avoided when possible (for example, wear rubber gloves when using cleaning chemicals, try not to inhale someone else's cigarette smoke), but many toxins cannot always be avoided. Toxic foods burden our cells and can wreak havoc on our bodies. Toxins that make it into our bodies, and are not eliminated, are stored in fat cells. This means that as the fat is released, so are the toxins.

Then what happens?

The fat and the toxins are processed by the liver. This means that during your fat loss journey, because of an overload of released toxins, the liver can become congested. This can slow down digestion and cause nausea, constipation, and tiredness.

So, what is a girl (or guy) to do?

Well, flushing (FYF4Good Pillar #6) is important to keep the liver, kidneys, and bladder clean. Also, detoxing (FYF4Good Pillar #5) is vital. Optimizing detoxing and clearing the body of the toxins is one of the most important benefits for the body to promote a feeling of health and well-being.

Another way that we protect the healthy cells is with good antioxidants. Antioxidants are found in fruits and vegetables, but as discussed previously, fruits and vegetables do not contain everything that they used to contain. Therefore, it is now wise to supplement with effective antioxidants.

Be careful when selecting an antioxidant supplement. Some of them are PRO-oxidative and cause damage to the body due to improper development of the supplement. Do your research before you swallow! When selecting an antioxidant, we want to protect both the fat and the water in the cells. You do not want a product that just protects the fat or just protects the water. And of course, make sure your choice is from whole-foods.

If you add five to seven fruits and vegetables per day to your Lifestyle, you will boost your antioxidant protection. That is good. In FYF4Good we are doing that because we eat a lot of healthy fruits and vegetables, two servings a day. But adding the right antioxidant supplement to this Lifestyle is highly recommended as you will be losing fat rapidly. Added protection for your cells is a GREAT benefit!

4) **Your endocrine system needs support!** You might ask "My *what* system?" Your endocrine system is made up of glands that secrete hormones directly into the circulatory system to message target organs. The main endocrine glands are the pineal and pituitary glands in the brain, thyroid gland, adrenal glands, pancreas, ovaries and testes. There are also other organs that have secondary endocrine functions which are the bone, liver, heart and kidneys. But every major organ and cell in your body is regulated by hormones. It is a very dynamic system to care for the functional demands of the body. In fact, the body uses eighty-seven hormones to function properly. Only seventeen hormones are sexually related.

What does that mean? That means hormones are extremely important for proper function of your body. Therefore, it is important that your endocrine system is supported and balanced as it is creating these hormones. Think **Phytosterols!**

In order to function properly, your endocrine system needs phytosterols from your Lifestyle. Phyto comes from a Greek word meaning plant. Sterols mean hormones. Phytosterols are plant hormones. Our bodies need them every day for the endocrine system to be supported and work at its best.

The human body needs from one to two grams of phytosterols a day. The modern diet provides only a fraction of that. *What?*

You heard it right … only a fraction of phytosterols are consumed daily in our modern diet. Ooops! Ever wonder why we are seeing a lot of cholesterol, thyroid, endocrine system problems in our society as well as PMS and male and female menopause issues? Additionally, if you are overfat, your hormones are probably in chaos. Losing the fat, while supplementing with a whole-food phytosterol supplement, has shown great benefit to help return balance and order to the endocrine system.

For optimum function of your organs, we recommend that you provide your body with the missing phytosterols that you are currently NOT getting. *Keep reading!*

5) **Make sure you have enough vitamin B12.** One concern around the world is the prevalence of a deficiency of B12. There is lack of food in some regions, poor eating habits, and aging which contribute to this concern. Vegans can develop the deficiency, as their diet lacks foods rich in B12 vitamins. Most commonly, with the reduction of gastric enzymes as we age, B12 absorption becomes impaired in the gut, especially those individuals sixty years old and over. And having a deficiency of B12 may cause an anemic condition called pernicious anemia which can be a significant health concern. As a result of the concern about the prevalence of the deficiency, you will see many ready-to-eat cereals "fortified with B12" in an effort to supplement synthetic B12 to the population in the food. Animal foods are the only natural source of vitamin B12. It is found naturally in fish, red meat, poultry, milk, and eggs. FYF4Good optimizes digestion, absorption and elimination, especially with Pillars #2 (Food Combining), #3 (Low-Glycemic Eating) and #4 (Nutrifying). Therefore, eating the FYF4Good way, most people do *not* experience a vitamin B12 deficiency.

6) **We need the right amount of enzymes for our digestive system**. Did you know that most people lose their digestive

enzyme forming capability as they age? Believe it or not, many people are NOT able to digest the foods or nutrients from the foods they are eating due to inadequate secretion of their own digestive enzymes. Why? Aging, inadequate nutrition, stress, and a hurried, over-worked lifestyle.

What does that mean? Your digestive enzymes are used in your stomach and throughout your gastrointestinal tract to break down your food for absorption. Your stomach does not have teeth. Part of the lesson to learn here is that you need to chew your food thoroughly before you swallow it. But chewing is not enough. Digestion in the stomach is a chemical process using enzymes. If you have fewer enzymes, your digestion will not work as efficiently.

Supplementing with high quality digestive enzymes is imperative, as it aids in optimal digestion to allow you to absorb your foods properly. Absorption is everything!

7) **Probiotics are necessary for our intestines**. Have you noticed that foods in the grocery stores are processed more than in years gone by? Part of that is good. We are successfully removing bad bacteria and other harmful impurities from our foods. But not all bacteria are bad for the human body. Along with the bad bacteria, we are removing the good bacteria.

Bacteria are used in the intestines to extract nutrition from our foods, as well as serving to increase the activity of the immune system. With every bowel movement, we lose approximately half of the good bacteria in our digestive tract. If we do not have enough good bacteria in our bodies, we are challenged to absorb enough of the nutrition that we need. That means that our bodies will signal us to eat more food to fill that void. And when we eat more food, we usually crave foods that give us sugar and starch because they boost our energy, which may be low due to nutritional deficiencies.

Live bacteria, when consumed in adequate amounts, helps promote your gastrointestinal health, aids in digestion, aids and strengthens the immune system and assists in nutrient absorption. FYF4Good is about DIGESTION, ABSORPTION and ELIMINATION.

When selecting a probiotic, you will notice that most are labeled with CFU. CFU stands for colony forming units—the higher the number, the better. Many probiotics are labeled with their CFU at manufacture. The number that you really want to know is their CFU at expiration. You want to know, if you take this on the expiration date, how many CFU can you expect to get into your digestive tract?

Did you know that 70 to 80 percent of your immune system is located in your digestive system? So, probiotic health in the gut serves a much larger benefit to our overall health than most people realize. Health is all about absorbing the nutrients you eat and having a strong immune system to handle any issues that arise.

Take your probiotic just before you go to bed, right before brushing your teeth. They will colonize overnight while you are sleeping, multiplying to provide *more* good bacteria in your intestines before you eat your fruit in the morning. You will be setting yourself up for good absorption of your nutrition starting at breaking your fast, (breakfast).

8) **There are supplements that can assist in fat loss**. FYF4Good recommends three supplements: Super Lean Aminos (Muscle Building-Fat Burning Powder), GLA (Gamma Linolenic Acid), and CLA (Conjugated Linoleic Acid).

The Most Important Supplements to Aid Fat Loss

First, we recommend taking FYF4Good Super Lean Aminos, a complex of amino acids, calcium and BCAAs (branch chain amino acids). Supporting and building your lean muscle mass is imperative to not only holding up your skeletal structure, but also helps in burning fat. Studies show that when you lose weight, the natural tendency of the human body is to lose half of that weight in fat and half in muscle and bone density. This makes yo-yo dieting especially hard on the body because when you stop the weight loss program and gain some weight back, the newly added weight is almost entirely fat, therefore putting fat back on fat. Not good!

Take an example of a person who loses twenty pounds. On the typical "diet," the person would lose ten pounds of fat and ten pounds of muscle and bone density. If they then go back to their former eating habits and gain back twenty pounds, most of that gain will be fat. They will now be worse off in terms of body composition than they were when they started the diet. Even their posture will change since their muscle tone and bone density is worse.

Second, we recommend GLA (Gamma Linolenic Acid) which contains Omega-3 and Omega-6 fatty acids to help with fat-burning. It is important to understand the nature of our body fat. Did you know that you have two types of fat on your body—brown fat and white fat? It was once thought that only babies have brown fat for protection against the cold. Brown fat helps babies, who do not yet have the ability to shiver to stay warm. But that theory was proved incorrect in 2009 when researchers found brown fat in adults.

Interestingly, they found that people with a lower body mass index tended to have more brown fat. Obese people have much less brown fat, sometimes insignificant amounts. This fat is called brown (or yellow) fat because of its color, which comes from iron and blood in the fat. The brown fat's ability to burn calories has sparked a huge interest in fighting the obesity epidemic. Unlike regular old white fat, which stores calories, mitochondria-packed brown fat cells burn for energy and produce heat.

Brown fat is found in unpredictable locations in the body. Although some brown fat is hard to find, as it is mixed up with the white fat, there are some trends on where to find it. One common place to find brown fat is in the neck and the shoulders region. Recently they have found brown fat in the chest and down the spines of healthy young men.

You will always have both kinds of fat. White fat stores excess calories. Brown fat generates heat and burns calories. When adults are exposed to cold temperatures, the brown fat may serve as an "internal heating blanket" to keep blood warm as it flows back to the heart and brain. People who are very overweight often do not have enough brown fat to burn the white fat.

There are several oils that are popular as supplements because they are high in fatty acids. **Borage oil** is derived from the seed of the plant Borago officinalis, also known as starflower. **Evening primrose oil** is derived from the yellow wildflower, Oenothera biennis. Both of these **oils** along with **black currant seed oil** are rich sources of gamma-linolenic acid (GLA). But not all omega-6 fatty acids are the same. We recommend **black currant seed oil** as it has two advantages over evening primrose oil and borage. In addition to omega-6 fatty acid, it has omega-3. We do not recommend borage oil because it might contain pyrroldizidine alkaloids, compounds that can damage the liver. We feel taking **black currant seed oil** is safer and a higher amount can be consumed.

Studies revealed that GLA supplementation had many of the following benefits:

> Stimulates brown fat activity through its prostaglandin pathways for optimized fat burning
>
> Supports healthy cholesterol levels
>
> Provides antioxidant properties
>
> Reduces excess inflammation and alleviates stiffness
>
> Provides excellent skin protection to moisturize internally and diminish symptoms of eczema and psoriasis
>
> Helps relieve PMS (pre-menstrual syndrome) in women

Third, we recommend the supplement **CLA,** short for **conjugated linoleic acid,** which supports and prompts the body to burn stored fat as energy. CLA is a naturally occurring critical fatty acid that we consumed in the past and was found in butter from grass-fed cows, raw dairy products from grass-fed cows, and red meats from animals that are grass-fed. Now, with our modern farming practices, most cows are grain-fed. As a result of this switch, our consumption of CLA has been reduced by 80 percent! CLA works by preventing the enlargement of your fat cells. It breaks up your fat cells, some of which are used to build lean muscle mass, and some are eliminated from the body. But CLA also targets the abdomen to help to get rid of that belly fat that often will not budge.

Studies revealed that CLA supplementation had many of the following benefits:

> **Reduced body fat** by up to 8 percent without changes in diet and exercise (reported in *International Journal of Obesity*)
> **Increased feelings of fullness** and decreased hunger (reported in the *European Journal of Clinical Nutrition*)
> **Maintains and increases lean muscle** mass (reported in *Journal of Nutrition*)
> **Supports healthy cholesterol levels**
> **Enhances immune function and anti-cancer effects** (reported in *The American Journal of Clinical Nutrition*)
> **Provides antioxidant properties**
> **Reduces body fat** (adiposity) and inflammation associated with it (reported in *The Journal of Nutritional Biochemistry*)
> **Reduces excess inflammation and alleviates stiffness**
> **Increased bone mass** in middle-aged female mice (reported in *Journal of Bone and Mineral Metabolism*)

FYF4Good recommends a CLA supplement for its many potential health benefits, but also to help win the battle of the bulge.

Recommended Supplement Shopping List

The FYF4Good team is always evaluating new supplements, reading studies, and taking the supplements ourselves. YES! We practice what we preach. We want to take the best of the best. We are happy to share with you our recommendations for high quality supplements, where to buy them, and the recommended amount to take. Visit our website at

FlushYourFat4Good.com and we will keep you updated with excellent options of what we have found. Do not rely on packaging, marketing gimmicks, or what your next-door neighbor is taking. You only have one body. Treat it like it is a valuable machine, because it is!

PILLAR #5

DETOXING

Sound the Trumpets! We Live in a Toxic World!

Why Do We Want to "Detox" Our Bodies?

Toxins are everywhere. We know this because we can see and smell it in our air (cigarette smoke, lead from cars, smog, fumes from farms or factory machinery, oil refinery omissions, paint fumes), our water (waste from our factories, dumping of oils and chemicals, flushing prescription drugs and urine loaded with medications down the toilet), our food (pesticides, weed killers, chemical additives, sugar, artificial colors or sweeteners, preservatives), our home environment (household cleaners, air fresheners, cheap pots and pans), the products we use (nail polish, skin care, makeup, lotions), medicine and synthetic supplements ... the list goes on and on. We breathe in toxins, we consume toxins, and we absorb toxins through the skin. It does not matter if we eat, drink, breathe, or touch them; a toxin is a toxin, and it will wreak havoc on and in our bodies. So, the first step is to avoid as many of them as possible.

Once in the body, toxins travel everywhere and do damage. It does not matter how they get in, the blood will pick up and move those toxins. When possible, the body will release them through our elimination systems. Our bodies were not made to recognize toxins as acceptable, and those toxins not released with body waste, are stored primarily in fat cells. Additionally, toxins can be deposited in many parts of our body and disrupt the health of our bones, blood, tissue, muscles, organs, and hormone functioning. Toxins make you feel lousy, clog up your digestive tract, cause headaches, make you feel lethargic, disrupt the function of your cells, affect your hormones, and can cause fatal diseases like cancer.

On FYF4Good when our body starts breaking down the fat for energy, the toxins will be released into the blood stream and carried to our liver and kidneys. We detox our bodies, moving the toxins through the liver, kidneys and colon out of the body. It is critical to get these out of our bodies if we want to achieve optimal health. This is why antioxidants and CranFlush are so important! By drinking lots of CranFlush, these toxins will be filtered out of the body 4Good. The antioxidants will help protect healthy cells from damage as the toxins are moving out of the body. If you add raw ginger juice to the CranFlush, it is helpful with inflammation that can be caused by the toxins and stress. We call it CranGingerFlush. Ginger is also an appetite suppressant, immune system modulator and has anti-cancer properties. It is so great for the digestive system and it increases your salivation making you want to drink more. Plus, it is delicious for all you ginger lovers.

As we keep everything moving through the body, we want to make sure we detox not only the liver and kidneys, but the colon! Years of poor eating, horrible digestion and constipation have clogged up the colon walls. Did you know that some people have fecal matter stuck on their colon walls? If you have suffered from long-term constipation, your colon could be impacted if you are not having regular bowel movements. YUCK. With all this build-up the beneficial nutrition that must be transported through the colon wall via the mucosa cells and the villi hairs, will have a hard time getting into the bloodstream. If it does not make it to the bloodstream, it will not be able to be absorbed and sent throughout the body for building, repairing, maintaining, and correcting your health.

Fruit is considered nature's "scrub brush" so always remember to eat at least two large servings every day, one first thing in the morning and one later on in the day. It will help to scrub clean those dirty colon walls. Seriously.

Be aware that some toxins will never be fully eliminated from our body. The preservative EDTA is a great example. We do not want to keep feeding our body more toxic chemicals while we are trying to eliminate them from the body. Please read labels on food and other products. Do not put those toxins in! And remember, *If God made it, EAT IT! If man made it, READ IT!*

Health Effects of Cow Dairy Products

If you have consumed your share of dairy products from cows, you may have mucus in your lungs and in your bowels. Cow milk has peptide chains, the cow's own hormones that are designed to take a calf into a one-ton animal with three stomachs. This is true regardless if the milk is organic or not. Most humans have a very hard time digesting dairy from a cow. You do not have to be diagnosed as lactose intolerant for this to be true. As a result, inflammation and irritation affects the human body by creating mucus. Most cow dairy is pasteurized instead of raw, which means it was heated to a very high temperature, and all the bacteria (good and bad) and enzymatic life has been cooked out of it. Therefore, it is a dead food. Eliminating cow dairy from your Lifestyle (and your children's Lifestyle), will improve your health and diminish and release that mucus from your body. Following the FYF4Good *Lifestyle to a "T"* will allow your body, through its innate intelligence, to automatically take care of this. For more information about cow dairy, see chapter nine: "FYF4GOOD Staples."

Yeast Overgrowth

There has been media attention and awareness given to yeast overgrowth in the body over the last twenty years due to the fact it is a very common infection. The most common strain is known as Candida Albicans. Usually present in the body in numbers that are under control, at times yeast can overgrow and wreak havoc. There are many reasons this will occur. The strength and effectiveness of the immune system and diet seem to be the two most important contributing factors. When the immune system is below 50 percent effective, the yeast starts to proliferate. Therefore, supporting your immune system is essential. Another common cause of yeast overgrowth is repeated rounds of antibiotics or extensive antibiotic therapy.

If you have been eating poorly for a long time, especially foods that contain sugar and starches made with white flour: bread, crackers, cookies, muffins, etc., there is a good chance your body has developed an overgrowth of yeast. Starch converts to sugar. Yeast thrives on sugar and vinegars. Avoid all fermented foods, sugars, and starches.

As you follow and eat according to the FYF4Good Phase 1 Lifestyle, the yeast will start to "die-off." By eliminating starches, vinegars and sugars the overgrowth of yeast will literally be starved out and killed. You may experience what is called a **Herxheimer Reaction**. The Herxheimer Reaction is a short-term (from days to weeks) detoxification reaction in the body. As the body detoxifies, it is not uncommon to experience flu-like symptoms including headache, joint and muscle pain, body aches, sore throat, general malaise, sweating, chills, nausea or other symptoms. There are several ways you might experience this. The skin is the largest organ of elimination so you may see a skin rash, on your torso, neck, chest, legs, back, in your arm pits, the folds of your body, or anywhere on your body. It will look red, may or may not itch, and may have a white shimmer on top. It also may be a very unusual looking rash. The good news is that it WILL resolve. But, if you have concerns about it, we recommend that you schedule an appointment with your health care practitioner to take a look at it.

Additionally, you may start experiencing loose stools, especially in the first several days of Phase 1. Your body will detox and flush the unwanted overgrowth of yeast as it is released and dies. As this is happening, you may experience severe cravings of sugar because yeast thrives on sugar. Please stay the course and trust the process of FYF4Good. Stay off the sugar now and forever. Protein will be your best friend along with immune support supplements. Maintaining consistent blood sugars by eating properly and consistently according to the recommendations throughout the day is also a key factor. Do not let yourself go far too long without eating or becoming really hungry. Try to eat when it is time to eat your next food group. These symptoms will disappear once the yeast has died-off. You will never completely eliminate all yeast from your body but having an overgrowth of yeast will compromise your health and immune system. So stay the course and get rid of the overgrowth! And, as always, should you have any concerns, please consult with your health care practitioner.

For more information about yeast overgrowth, refer to chapter ten: "Troubleshooting for Good Results."

Eating Organic Produce

One of the best things we could all do to minimize toxins, is to always try to eat organic produce. Pesticides on fruits and vegetables are something that is too easy to consume. Always remember to thoroughly clean your fruits and vegetables before eating. Additional factors, such as times of the year, where you live, and travel (especially traveling abroad), may make it difficult for you to eat organic foods, but do the best you can.

In 2013, the US Department of Agriculture (USDA) tested 3,015 produce samples for pesticide contamination. About two-thirds of the samples contained pesticide residues. The Environmental Working Group (EWG), a nonprofit, nonpartisan advocacy group for human health and environment, found a total of 165 different pesticides in this sampling by the USDA. Fruits like apples, peaches, and nectarines should ALWAYS be eaten organic as 100 percent of fruits tested had pesticide residue. But, there is good news. There are many non-organic fruits and vegetables that are safe to eat! Those fruits and vegetables with thick skins and are not conducive to pests, are safe to eat conventionally.

If you start experiencing burning of the tissues in your mouth, it may be the pesticides coming thru your mucus membranes as you detox. Double up on the CranFlush or lemon in water to get through this. Make sure you are nutrifying your body as you will be helping your cells cleanse, detoxify and repair. Do not buy fruits, vegetables, nuts, meats, or anything else produced in countries that have poor standards for regulating food safety. Be active in the Flush Your Fat 4Good "Buddies" Facebook Group where the latest information about foods is shared by our Buddies and Coaches. Protect yourself, and try to buy the very best from countries that have governments that strictly enforce regulatory practices in food safety.

Ultimately, your organs are responsible for detoxifying your body. To keep them performing at the optimal level, we must eat food that is as chemical and pesticide-free as much as possible. Your body will succumb to toxicity, but the great thing about burning and flushing fat is that we can expose those hidden toxins, and through the FYF4Good Lifestyle, we can effectively get many of them out of our body once and for all! This alone is going to improve your well-being and your health.

A Word About GMO

Genetically modified foods were designed by man to prolong their shelf life and eliminate the need for pesticides. With some GMO grown crops, when insects eat the plant, their stomach explodes, and they die. For the human body, we are not aware of all the damage that could result from eating GMO foods. Therefore, do not eat GMO foods. Countries are gradually outlawing GMO products, and hopefully this will continue. At the time of writing this book there are around thirty-eight countries, including Mexico, the Netherlands, Italy, Germany, Greece, and Belize, that ban GMOs. Many more have restrictions on GMOs. States like Hawaii also ban GMO foods. FYF4Good takes this seriously and recommends only non-GMO foods.

So remember: Clean your food thoroughly before eating and eat organic and vine-ripened fruits and vegetables whenever possible. Keep hydrated and avoid coming in contact with pesticides and chemicals. Through time your body will become cleaner and cleaner.

Your cells all have a lifespan. Each kind of cell will make a copy of itself before its lifespan is up. Each time your cells make copies, they will be healthier, stronger and better copies. The life of a red blood cell is about four months. The life of skin cells is ten to thirty days. Your DNA regenerates in two months, the brain will regenerate in one year. You will turn over your bones every three months and in seven to eight years you will have a whole new body including your fat cells. Every generation will create a newer, better YOU if you are feeding yourself correctly. If you move to a sterile environment, it will take about one year of clean eating and following the FYF4Good *Lifestyle to a "T"* and consistently nutrifying your body and drinking your CranFlush for the body to detox as much as possible. Since a sterile environment is not possible, Phase 2 of FYF4Good (clean eating, low or high-glycemic non-GMO fruits and vegetables, proper food combining, nutrifying, CranFlush) will continue to detox your body for the rest of your life.

Detox, Detox, Detox!

PILLAR #6

FLUSHING

The Pipes of Life

When was the last time you had a conversation with someone about POOP? How many times a day do you have a bowel movement? What did it look like? What size and consistency was it? What color was it? Did you have to strain to eliminate it? Are you taking stool softeners?

For most people, this is a very uncomfortable conversation to have. We do not talk about it. It is embarrassing. Often times we feel ourselves laugh uncomfortably if the topic is brought up.

The truth of the matter is we NEED to talk about it. FYF4Good is about digestion, absorption and ELIMINATION (Flushing). The bottom line is you better care about what hits that toilet bowl and how often it happens. Seventy to eighty percent (70 to 80 percent) of your immune system is in your gut. It is imperative to pay attention to your bowels (and critical to teach this to your children!)

If you have been eating poorly (junk food, bad fats, sugar, toxic preservatives), mis-combining foods, not supplementing your body with whole-food sourced vitamins and minerals, not taking digestive enzymes and probiotics, chances are what is hitting that toilet bowl is not what it should be. You may be only pooping once a day or maybe every other day. This could lead quickly to needing assistance with medication or enemas to clean your colon. This is not optimal health.

And guess what— you are not alone! If you were to have an open conversation with your close family and friends, I bet you will find a significant number of them have some kind of digestive issue.

Do you watch TV? If yes, have you ever stopped to think about how many commercials you see for constipation, irritable bowel syndrome, diarrhea, acid reflux, upset stomach? I bet if you flip the TV on right now you will not have to wait very long to see someone wrestling with a pizza slice or a bacon strip and recommending an OTC (over the counter) medication. Next time you are in the drug store check out how many different products they sell for these types of issues. Why? Because most of us have been eating incorrectly for so long that we now need products to try to offset the reaction of our bodies to what we are swallowing. This should be a crime! What are we doing to our bodies?

The majority of these conditions can be reversed by feeding your body the way God had intended it to be fed. Thousands of people that are living the FYF4Good Lifestyle are now enjoying optimal digestion, absorption and ELIMINATION! Yes, you too will enjoy the process of elimination once it is working correctly!

When one starts on FYF4Good, within a very short window of time your body will start to run smoother and more efficiently, digest foods effectively, and heal. And as a result, you will feel better. Some changes happen fast (inches start coming off, you start sleeping better, joints do not ache as much). But other changes happen more slowly, and you may not even know they are happening. The immune system prioritizes when changes take place. If you are well and have no issues, most likely you will have faster results. But make no mistake about it, *You Can Never Go Wrong Eating Right!* and your body knows that!

After a short time on FYF4Good you may start to have a little constipation. Do not be alarmed. This is what we call a congested or compromised liver from the toxins coming out of the fat cells and filtered through the liver. Toxins harbor in the fat cells for years and many are dangerous. Drink extra CranFlush, get in at least three big servings of low-glycemic fruit (at the proper times, do not mis-combine) and everything will start to move along normally within a few days. The constipation is an indicator you are breaking down FAT! The toxins must be filtered from your body. Ride it out and you will watch those pounds and inches shed off your body. An extra digestive enzyme supplement before protein meals, and an extra probiotic at bedtime will help. If constipation is really severe, visit FlushYourFat4Good.

com for recommended supplements or see your health care practitioner to make sure there is not something additional to be concerned about.

Let's talk about POOP … baby!

Other than "feeling better," how can you tell if your body is optimally digesting and absorbing the foods and nutrients you are feeding it? There is no quick test you can do to measure this, but the changes you will start to see in your bowel movements are a great indicator for how well your digestive system is working. Stool analysis is an extremely common diagnostic tool used by health care professionals. So take a closer look at your fecal matter. You heard me right!

Length

The optimal length of a bowel movement should be about ten to twelve inches. If it is significantly shorter, such as shaped in round pellets, this may indicate constipation. Constipation can occur for a number of reasons, one of which is liver congestion. Increasing your dietary fiber intake and staying hydrated will help. That is why when following the FYF4Good Lifestyle we eat a lot of low-glycemic fruits and vegetables and drink lots of CranFlush!

Width

The width of your bowel movement should be about the width of your thumb (two centimeters). If your stool starts to become consistently narrow, you should consult with your health care practitioner. Thinning bowel movements may indicate an obstruction in your large intestines such as a foreign object or a tumor. Do not panic but get it checked out as soon as possible. If your stool is wider, that is fine, unless you are straining.

Consistency

Your bowel movement should be smooth, solid, and a little fluffy. If it breaks apart easily or is mostly liquid, of course that is diarrhea. Diarrhea can be caused by a wide range of health problems including:

Infectious disease
Inflammation

Nutrient malabsorption
Psychological stress
Food poisoning
Yeast "die-off"

Yeast "die-off" can happen as early as one to two days after starting FYF4Good and then periodically thereafter. One of the benefits of Phase 1 eating is to reduce the amount of yeast in your body. Phase 1 is the best way to manage and correct yeast overgrowth.

Bowel movements that are lumpy, hard, extra wide, and difficult to pass indicate constipation. As we know, this can be very uncomfortable. To relieve the discomfort, elevate your feet on a step stool. If your knees are higher than your bottom, your rectum will be able to more effectively evacuate the stool completely, for a more comfortable bowel movement. If you are in a public restroom, or otherwise do not have access to a step stool, place your left ankle on your right knee. The last portion of your large intestine or descending colon, before the rectum and anus, is on the left side of your body, so having the left side of your body in alignment is especially helpful. Sounds weird, but TRY IT!

Your Poop Should Sink. Listen for the sound of your **stool** as it hits the water in the toilet. **Floating stools** are often an indication of high fat or high fiber content, a change of foods resulting in more gas into your digestive system, a sign of malabsorption, or a sign of an intestinal infection.

Frequency

Believe it or not, the vast majority of people go days without having a decent bowel movement. This is not good. Remember upwards to 80 percent of the immune system is in the digestive tract. If the digestive tract is backed up, we are more likely to get sick or have real health problems. You should be moving your bowels two to three times PER DAY minimum! If you do not, the poop sits there while the colon keeps absorbing the water out of it and you are left with very hard stools or constipation! As it stays in the colon for too long, you will begin to absorb toxins that should be eliminated. Additionally, your appetite will diminish, and you will feel bloated. You do not want any of these results.

When you have been on FYF4Good for a while, you will start to notice that most of your bowel movements happen in the morning. This is the rhythm of the body, the circadian rhythm. Our bodily function from 4:00 a.m. until 12:00 p.m. noon is ELIMINATION, which is why fruit first thing in the morning is beneficial. *Fruit is "nature's scrub brush."* During the night, your digestive tract has been processing and moving things along, so you will be ready to eliminate in the morning. Therefore, the best time to take probiotics is right before your head hits the pillow. The probiotics will colonize throughout the night, and in the morning they will be ready to receive the nutrition (fruit) you will be sending down to them the whole rest of the day.

Stool Color
The ideal color of your stool is medium brown. You, of course, may see variations and when you do, this is a great time to ask yourself why that is happening.

- **Green or Yellow** usually indicates the bowels are moving too fast, as with mild diarrhea. Bile is the main pigment in poop. It starts out yellow, becomes green if blood is introduced, and turns to brown overtime. So, if you see green or yellow poop, that is an indicator it is moving through your body too quickly and is classified as diarrhea.

- **Pale Grey or Yellow or White** may indicate liver disease, including hepatitis or cirrhosis (scarring) of the liver. The liver is an amazing organ. It is a sponge for the body. It regenerates itself if damaged and filters one point four (1.4) liters of blood per minute. It is believed that the liver has one million functions but one of its main functions is to detoxify the colon. If you are ***consistently*** seeing pale grey or yellow or white, make an appointment with your health care practitioner!

- **Red** may indicate there is blood in your stool. Pay attention to any stool that is red. **Bright red** may indicate bleeding late in the digestive tract, likely the large intestine or anus. Many times this is a non-serious health issue. Maybe minor inflammation, hemorrhoids, or a rectal fissure (a tear that usually heals easily but can be painful—often caused by constipation). In rare cases, bright red blood could indicate cancer. See your health care practitioner if you are seeing blood in your stool.

Red can also indicate that beets were eaten recently. Red-colored stools after eating beets looks different from the red color of blood. **And magenta or fuchsia**-colored stools are probably from food coloring.

- **Extremely dark red or black** (or a stool that is sticky or tar-like) may indicate bleeding higher up, in the stomach or small intestines. If you pass this type of stool, you really must talk to your health care practitioner. This could be something more serious like peptic ulcers or cancer. Bleeding higher up in the stomach, for example such as in a bleeding ulcer, may appear in your stools like coffee grounds in the toilet.

    If you eat A LOT of blackberries or blueberries, your stool may appear **black.** This does not mean you are bleeding, it just means you ate A LOT of blackberries or blueberries. The color should return to normal in a day or two (depending on how much you ate and over what period of time). (The same is true with A LOT of carrots and the color orange.)

Try not to be alarmed by other odd colors in your stool unless they persist. Food colorings can change the color of the bowel movement. We do not eat processed food on FYF4Good, so there should be no food coloring eaten; however, if food coloring was consumed before starting, or by mistake, it could show up.

Even if you do not see dyes in food, it may be hidden or masked by other colors. Mixing with other pigments during digestion may cause the bowel movement to be a different color than expected. Also, dyes mixed with the green or yellow bile can create interesting colors.

If there is a difference in color (from medium brown) that is consistent over time or you have any concerns whatsoever, please do not hesitate to consult with your health care practitioner to rule out any issues you may have.

What About Flatulence? How Does That Happen?

Digestion in the stomach is activated by heat, acid and enzymes. If you do not combine your food properly (i.e. you "mis-combine"), you may have bloating, indigestion, and possibly bowel pain or cramps. When food just "sits" in your stomach, not digesting, you will get gas. Conversely, if you are due to eat your next meal, you may also experience gas. This is especially true if you are sensitive to yeast overgrowth. Yeast will grow with a rise or drop in blood sugar. So make sure you are eating and not skipping a meal.

For proper health, it is essential to have a clean, functioning liver. When following the FYF4Good Lifestyle (including taking the supplements, following the way we eat, and consuming the CranFlush), your liver will clear out and function better. After a year on FYF4Good, the digestive tract will be cleaner!

Flushing Your Urinary Tract

Flushing on FYF4Good also refers to keeping your urinary tract clean and in good working order. Hydration is key here! Your liver and your kidneys process toxins as they are released from your fat cells. If you have a lot of fat to lose, that means a lot of toxins will be on the move. If your kidneys and bladder do not receive enough liquids, you can develop an infection in your urinary tract, or even worse, kidney stones. Make sure you are getting your minimum recommended amount of CranFlush on a daily basis for optimal urinary tract health! By the way, you can also have water after you have met your daily quota of the CranFlush. Squeezing juice from one half of a lemon in your water is also excellent.

Do Not Worry!

Follow the FYF4Good *Lifestyle to a "T"* and you will start seeing your digestive system get healthier and healthier. Many people have discovered that their digestive tract was never working correctly. For some, it may take a few weeks to get the digestive tract back on track, for others several months. But it WILL happen!

One of the best pieces of advice Jackie's dad ever gave her: "Look before you flush!"

PILLAR #7

EXERCISE & SLEEP

Exercise

We have ALL been misled. You do NOT need to spend three hours a day in the gym running at full speed, riding a bike at one hundred RPMs, nor doing hard core group aerobics, to get the pounds off. Number one; who has time to do that? Number two; this will not happen if you are significantly overweight. Strenuous exercise such as this is not possible for some people, and according to global studies, not necessary.

Brisk walking, while swinging your arms, is one of the most beneficial exercises you can do.... So that is exactly what we recommend on FYF-4Good. Thirty to forty-five minutes (not stopping), five days a week, is your way to better health. One hundred fifty minutes minimum per week is recommended. And guess what? There are global studies showing this is the optimal exercise to improve health and prolong life. You of course can do more exercise than this, and you will receive benefit from it.

What does walking do for your body?

- Boosts endorphins; eases stress, tension, depression, anger, fatigue, and confusion
- Cuts in half the odds of getting a cold
- Decreases appetite by decreasing blood sugar through a mechanism that does not involve insulin
- Works your arms and shoulder muscles, as you swing your arms while walking

- Strengthens your leg and abdominal muscles including: quadriceps, hip flexors, and hamstrings
- Builds lean muscle mass
- Builds bone mass, reducing the risk of osteoporosis
- Reduces glaucoma risks
- If you walk regularly for five years, it cuts in half the risk of Alzheimer's
- Improves heart health by increasing circulation
- Increases metabolism
- Reduces the risk of colon cancer by 31 percent for women
- Improves balance
- Strengthens your overall core
- Burns belly fat
- Walking for exercise early in the day tricks the brain to think it is time to burn fat when you walk for any time the rest of the day

Just DO IT! What do you have to lose? ☺

If walking is stressful on your joints because of your current weight or for other health reasons, get into a swimming pool! We are seeing amazing results from our FYF4Good Power100 Heroes (one hundred or more pounds to lose) who are diving right in! The water in a swimming pool will take the stress off your painful joints by removing gravity. For most people, this will allow you to move pain-free. It will also provide resistance, so the faster you start moving in the pool, the quicker that blood is going to be moving through your body and carry needed oxygen and nutrition to your bones, blood, tissue, muscles, and organs. No matter what weight you are, if you have painful joints, swimming is a great option.

If you are confined to your home, start with what you can do. Walking in place is fine. If you cannot walk, then move your arms or your legs in a consistent way five to ten times. Twist your body from side to side five to ten times. If you have a helper, have them help you to get to the edge of the bed so that they can help you to stand with a walker then sit down and do it again. Repeat up to three to five times depending on your size and capability. Work up to thirty to forty-five minutes continually moving without stopping, but do not get discouraged if the first day you can only do five minutes. If you can only walk around your house for ten minutes, do it! Each week gradually increase the length of time. It will not take long to build on this as long as you are consistent. You must get your body moving, in whatever way you can, and progress will be made.

If you are bedridden, there are exercises that you can do while lying down. Do circular motions with your feet, legs, and arms, in a repetitive fashion. Write each letter of the alphabet pointing your big toe, first the right foot, then the left foot. Invest in inexpensive resistance bands and overtime, as your muscles strengthen, add ankle and wrist weights to your routine. Begin with light weights. The goal is to strengthen the muscles, and the more muscle you have, the faster you burn the fat. The key to satisfy the exercise Pillar is ACTIVITY. So, do what you can, until you can do more!

The Big Myth

"You do not start burning fat until you are twenty minutes into your workout." WRONG!

Muscle burns a combination of fat and carbohydrates (glucose) simultaneously almost all the time. You may burn a higher percentage of one or the other, depending on the intensity of exercise. For example, when you do a heavy intensity workout, (sprinting, heavy weightlifting, hard cardio), you may be burning as much as 80 to 90 percent carbohydrates and only 10 percent fat.

At rest and with light intensity to brisk walking, the percentage changes to 70 percent fat and 30 percent carbohydrates. If you want to lose the fat, do not exercise at a pace where it is difficult to breathe or carry on a conversation.

Why is oxygen so important?

Fat requires a lot of oxygen to burn. If you cannot catch your breath while you are exercising, you will not be able to push the oxygen to your muscles. Your muscles will be forced to burn the carbohydrates, which come from your food, for fuel.

As you start to exercise, both fat and carbohydrates are released from storage sites in the body, as well as from the blood stream, and they enter the working muscle to be used for energy.

Why does your muscle prefer fat? Fat contains nine calories per gram. Carbohydrates have only four calories per gram. Your muscles prefer fat because it is so energy dense. Also, we are trying to lose fat. So, get enough oxygen in, and your muscles will burn it!

Think smart! Work smart! Not hard!

Once you have started burning through that fat, your body is working efficiently, and you have the FYF4Good Lifestyle down to a "T" you can start to push it a little: Walk, run, walk, run. This gives your body short bursts of intense energy and is great for fat burning. Other exercises people love to do are: resistance exercises using resistance bands, a NordicTrack, Total Gym, or weight training. Gardening, swimming and cleaning the house (like a maniac) are also *additional* exercises, but we recommend you still WALK!

Important Exercise Studies

In April 2015 a large-scale study was done to look at "How much exercise is too little, too much, or just right to improve health and longevity?" The researchers wanted to know if "extreme" exercise was harmful. SPOILER ALERT!! They found out this was "unlikely to be harmful."

But what else did they find? Any amount of exercise movement is better than none. Just get up and move. Exercise reduces the risks of many diseases and pre-mature death. Did you ever hear the saying "If you don't use it, you lose it"? Think about what happens if you are confined to a bed or wheelchair. Your muscles atrophy, they shrink up because they are not being used. A muscle will grow when it is being used. The same thing goes for your heart, which is a very important muscle.

At the time of the study, current government regulations recommend one hundred fifty (150) minutes moderate exercise to build and maintain health and fitness. Thirty minutes, five times a week was the baseline.

The results of the study were published in the *Journal of American Medical Association* (JAMA) Internal Medicine. Researchers with the National Cancer Institute at Harvard University, along with many other institutions, gathered and pulled data on peoples' exercise habits from six large ongoing health surveys. This totaled over 661,000 adults, most middle aged.

Using the data, researchers tracked these adults based upon the amount of time they exercised: those that did not work out at all to below the recommended amount, those that worked out at a moderate amount (the recommended 150 minutes) per week, and those that exercised twenty-five hours per week (three-and-one-half hours per day, seven days a week...ten times the recommended amount!) Again, they wanted to see if "extreme" exercise was damaging to the body. They compared fourteen years of death records for this group.

Here are the findings about the effects of exercising on our body:

- People who did not exercise had the highest risk of early death. If you do not move, everything will slow down, including your heart and your lungs.

- Those who exercised a little (not meeting the requirements of 150 minutes per week but just doing something), lowered their risk of premature death by 20 percent. Think about how easy this is to do.

- The group that met the guidelines of 150 minutes per week, enjoyed greater health benefits and reduced their risk of premature death by 31 percent!

- The group that worked out three times the recommended amount, 450 per week, reduced their risk of premature death by 39 percent compared to those who did not exercise.

- After this, the benefits plateaued, but did not reduce. So those that were extreme, exercising ten times higher than the recommended guidelines of 150 minutes did not increase or decrease their risk. Their risk is equal to those working out at three times the recommended amount.

Conclusion: Moderation in exercise is the key!

There are other very large studies, one based in Australia looking at 200,000 people and confirming that meeting the 150 minutes of required exercise substantially reduced the risk of early death. It also confirmed that if someone engaged occasionally in vigorous exercise, it gave them a little more benefit.

An important point here is these large studies are occurring on different continents, but are showing very similar results, eliminating environmental factors.

Remember that fat is the premium fuel. Exercise is required to replace fat with lean muscle. Exercise keeps the fat burning, increases metabolism and circulation, and facilitates detoxing and flushing. Exercise is extremely important to lessen the chances of premature death.

Sleep

Why is sleep included in the same Pillar as Exercise? The answer is very simple. Even when people do not get enough sleep, they will often force themselves to go out walking or to the gym. They may keep pushing themselves day after day to get that exercise in. What they fail to acknowledge is that sleep is just as important as exercise for losing fat. Additionally, both the quality and the quantity of your sleep are important and will have a huge impact on how you lose fat. Sleep has also been shown to "reset" or "reboot" the brain, which is another great benefit that plays in to all the vast functions of the brain. If you are not seeing the fat loss results you expect to see, perhaps you should ask yourself the question: *How am I sleeping?*

Let's Dig Further

Lack of sleep increases daytime cortisol levels. Cortisol is a hormone released in the body that works to break down muscle and increase fat. If you have a lot of stress, cortisol levels are high in your body. This signals the fight or flight mechanism in our body and we begin to put on reserves, extra fat.

In one study from The Laboratory of Physiology in Belgium, research showed those who were shorting their periods of sleep had higher afternoon and early evening cortisol levels than those who were not.

One study in Chicago noted that ongoing sleep deprivation is responsible for change in the hormonal release and metabolism in humans. You will have an increase in hunger and appetite. You will crave sugars and starches because of having low energy and being fatigued from lack of sleep. It kick-starts your craving to eat. If you are always hungry, ask yourself the question: "Am I getting enough sleep?"

Decreased sleep may increase glucose and reduce insulin sensitivity. This is not good! The amount of sleep is critical in development (or prevention) of diabetes, as well as regulating the satiety. Satiety tells your body it is full and should stop eating.

Sleep is extremely important when it comes to your health. For example, if you only get four to five hours of sleep on a regular basis, your risk for diabetes dramatically increases. There are rare incidences of people only needing four to five hours, but that is not the norm. Additionally, sleep increases growth hormones (GH) in your body. Growth hormone help you stay thinner and leaner and aids in repair and regeneration of human tissue. Your GH levels at age thirty are about 20 percent of what they were in childhood. GH declines 12 to 15 percent per decade after thirty.

So how does "sleep" affect the two different types of fat?

Visceral adipose tissue (visceral fat) is the most important fat to lose because it sets you up for the greatest overall health threats. Visceral fat is wrapped around the internal organs in the main cavities of the body, especially the abdomen, and is much more difficult to get rid of. Because it is around the organs, you cannot see where it is when looking in a mirror. You cannot liposuction it out either.

Excess visceral fat is life-threatening! Recent studies show soft drinks increase your visceral fat. We do not want this! If you have a lot of visceral fat you may experience sleep apnea as the fat crowds out your visceral organs. It can crowd your heart and lungs to the degree where they cannot expand or contract correctly. IMAGINE THIS!

Subcutaneous fat is more noticeable, our body puts it on faster, and you can see it. It is the fluffy looking fat just under the skin. It is easy to measure the changes in subcutaneous fat when you are adding or losing fat. A simple tape measure will do.

Sleep Studies

Researchers from John Carroll University used a continuous dark versus a continuous light exposure, testing the impact on animals. They measured the melatonin levels, metabolic parameters, circadian rhythm, as well as any behavior changes, different from those animals in a twelve-hour light, twelve-hour dark condition.

The animals that experienced twenty-four hours light had increased deposits of visceral adipose tissues (dangerous fat), had a lower level of activity, and became extremely irritable and very excitable verses the other two groups that had darkness.

Conclusion: The body wants to maintain a normal circadian rhythm with the proper balance of light and darkness, and seven to eight hours of sleep. When these are altered, negative effects (increased fat, decreased overall health) start to happen to the body.

In Czechoslovakia, a study published in *Physiology Research* found that optimal body weight is strongly associated with seven hours of sleep. If you get seven hours of continuous sleep, the weight that your body maintains will be optimal.

If you have difficulty getting to sleep or do not sleep well, you could have a number of issues that are interfering with this: stress, adrenals, mis-combining of food. If you are waking up in the middle of the night, perhaps you did not have enough exercise during the day or you did not eat enough protein throughout the day to maintain your blood sugar. Hormonal balance could also be a factor, so we encourage nutrifying with more of the food supplement containing phytosterols that will allow your body to balance the hormones naturally. Try doubling your intake of the recommended phytosterols supplement. We eat and nutrify on FYF4Good to keep the body rapidly burning the stored fat for fuel and to create homeostasis, which is a healthy balance.

If you still have sleeping issues, talk to your Buddy or Coach, ask questions in the Facebook Group or dial in on a live support call. If you still need a safe, natural, drugless solution try:

- Valerian Root: 450 mg 2X a night
- Melatonin: 5 mg to 10 mg
- Tryptophan together with the co-factors (B6 or pyridoxyl-5-phosphate) releases serotonin that relaxes your brain and promotes sleep.

- A cup of hot milk (recommended milk only) with the FYF4Good Super Lean Aminos (Muscle Building-Fat Burning Powder) whisked in with it. This can relax you and the added protein will help you to sleep.

Take one of these twenty minutes before bedtime, preferably on an empty stomach. You do not have to do it forever. Take it during the week of going on daylight savings time if you are one who experiences sleep disturbances during these changes. You may also want to take these natural supplements if you travel across different time zones.

Did you know that melatonin was developed as a sleep aid and was later discovered to be helpful for jet lag? It supports the pineal gland in the brain which responds to the circadian rhythm. It takes some people three weeks to get back on track after these disruptions.

Remember How Important Sleep Is

Sleep is like "money in the bank." It is extremely important to help you protect your very important asset, your HEALTH! Most Buddies report that sleep is one of the first noticeable improvements on following the recommendations of FYF4Good. Good, long, deep, restful, healing sleep—every night— is vital to your health. You cannot "catch up." Sweet Dreams!

PILLAR #8

SUPPORT & ACCOUNTABILITY

Why you won't feel discouraged and alone!

No skipping Pillar #8. This is one of the most important Pillars of this Lifestyle. If you are like most people who have fat to lose, you have tried one "diet" after another. You may have dropped some weight the first few weeks, or the first month with those programs, but then right back on it came—plus some extra. You most likely were disappointed, felt like a failure, and/or extremely frustrated that you worked so hard and went backward rather than forward. Your past experiences have been the never-ending yo-yo up and down, but mostly an upward climb of your weight. You have doubt as you read this and are saying to yourself, "This probably will not work for me, just like the rest."

With FYF4Good, you will only go forward to reach your goal of a lean and healthy body! This is *A Lifestyle for a Lifetime* and you are now on the road to better health in addition to melting that fat forever. If you are like most people, you want to just get started ... like yesterday! You want it simple and you want it to work quickly. Well guess what? FYF4Good is simple and it will work quickly, and through this you will be completely changing your relationship with food. As you interact with other Buddies on this journey, you will be encouraged in your own journey!

By embracing Pillar #8: Support & Accountability, you will have access to: coaching; live support calls (including a FYF4Good Power100 Heroes support call) most often hosted with the creators, Jackie Padgette-Baird and Dr. Victoria Arcadi and special Coaches that have lost over one hundred pounds; an incredibly supportive and *PRIVATE* Flush Your Fat 4Good "Buddies" Facebook Group; the FlushYourFat4Good. com website; archived support calls; and so much more right at your fingertips when you need it. Check FlushYourFat4Good.com for support opportunities.

It may be as simple as a quick question on finding where to buy goat yogurt when you are traveling… to "I am in the super market and really want to buy this tub of ice cream. HELP!" We are here for you 24/7, but you need to take the first step to connect. This is a very special community, a culture of caring and amazingly kind, supportive, and helpful Buddies and Coaches that only want the best for everyone. There is no competition here. And most importantly, you will have access to ALL the knowledge you will need to be successful. We are constantly updating the information as new studies and information about living healthy becomes available!

You are always one click away, one text away, one post away from the FYF4Good Buddies and Coaches who all want you to succeed! Over the years, some people have embraced Pillar #8, while others have avoided it. By far, those who embrace it are *much* more likely to be successful with this Lifestyle and see results much faster. Every aspect of this Pillar has been carefully planned. *You will not find a more caring and supporting group of Buddies anywhere on the planet!* Period. But in order to succeed, you have to participate!

How This Pillar Works:
The *Private* Flush Your Fat 4Good *"Buddies"* Facebook Group
Go to FlushYourFat4Good.com and learn how to join the private Facebook Group. This is the most important place to get connected and become part of the FYF4Good Community! As we are writing this book, over thirteen hundred Buddies are in the private group and there are over one hundred Global Certified FYF4Good Coaches. You will also be able to pick the brains of Dr. Vicky and Jackie who are very available in the Facebook Group.

No one can see your posts, except those who have been screened and added to the room. Everyone has skin in the game and they joined the community as a gesture of commitment. The room is positively monitored by administrators. This has kept the room a safe, private haven to post anything related to your journey that could be potentially embarrassing such as your weight, your pictures, your measurements, your fears, your weaknesses, or your successes. It is all good as everyone learns from these posts.

This is a global, twenty-four hours a day, seven days a week, three hundred sixty-five days a year support system that travels with you. When you have a question or concern, post in the group and within minutes you will have ten, twenty, or fifty people answering your questions and offering helpful tips.

If you are in the grocery store, about to make a poor choice on a food purchase, send out a *May Day* message and we will send some encouragement into your ear to make the right decision ("STEP AWAY FROM THE CHOCOLATE! STEP AWAY!").

You are safe in this room and you can private message anyone in the room to get the answer to your question. The Facebook Group is also where you will find your Buddies! What is a Buddy? Please read on!

Buddy-Up

You are changing the rest of your life. Why walk this path alone? The Flush Your Fat 4Good "Buddies" Facebook Group is a great place to get questions answered or see the amazing results of others. But, there will be times when you may need some extra encouragement, would like to share something personal, or just want to make this journey more fun by having friends on it with you.

How do you get a Buddy?

- Ask your spouse, boyfriend, girlfriend, neighbor, immediate family, relatives and/or friends to join FYF4Good so that you can all do it together. This is the absolute best way to have someone special in your life share this journey and to support each other. Whether it is shopping together, measuring each other, planning holiday meals that work with Phase 1, having a coffee or sharing a meal together, a close partner and Buddy is *very* effective. This is powerful because you have someone watching your back, and it makes this journey a lot more fun!

- If you learned about FYF4Good from someone living the Lifestyle, ask them to be your Buddy.
- Post on the private Facebook Group that you need a Buddy. You will be amazed at how many responses you get from those ready to help.

Decide how you will keep in touch with each Buddy. Through regular phone calls, text messages, Facebook instant messenger, carrier pigeon, or smoke signals. It is up to you, but have a plan.

What is a Buddy?

A *teacher*, when you have a question or need to know where to go to learn more

A *cheerleader*, when you have results to celebrate or need some encouragement

A *confidant*, someone you can share your personal story with

A *motivator*, when you do not seem to find the time to exercise

A *voice of reason*, to stop you in your tracks, when you want that candy bar

A *consoler*, if you need to cry

A *friend*

Your *partner* in this journey

You can have more than one Buddy or Coach, and in return you are also their Buddy. The more the merrier! And do not forget, all of the Buddies and Coaches in the Facebook Group are your Buddies dedicated to your success. This is so important. You will never find a more supportive, selfless, giving community.

In the beginning, set up regular calls with your Buddy, possibly daily, for the first fourteen to thirty days. Keep in touch until you are on automatic with this Lifestyle. It will not take long, but be honest with your Buddy. Let them help you succeed! There is no embarrassment or shame here. We have all been where you are.

Live Support Call(s)

There are multiple weekly support calls. This is your place to ask questions, report your results, and have someone coach you through your day if you think you might not be doing things quite right. Sometimes you just want things explained further, or you have several questions you want to talk through. Get on any one of the support calls and ask your questions. Visit our website at FlushYourFat4Good.com to learn how to join the support calls. You can count on the creators of this Lifestyle (Dr. Vicky and Jackie), a trained FYF4Good Coach or two, or a combination of these, will always be running the calls.

FYF4Good Power100 Heroes Support Call

This is a special call for our Buddies with around one hundred or more pounds to lose. FYF4Good specializes in Globesity. Obesity is a global issue and it is one we are passionate about! Everyone is welcome on this call, of course, as it is helpful for all. However, the call is focused on our Buddies with one hundred or more pounds to lose. This is specifically targeted for physical and emotional struggles, obesity related health issues, and questions that are unique to people with a tremendous amount of fat to lose. There are certain issues, emotional and physical, that are unique to people who feel that their fat loss is an impossible task, feeling that they will never get back to normal weight. This is a safe place to share about these struggles, and a place where you will realize you are not alone! This is a place to identify your old paradigms around eating, address why you have them, and redefine new paradigms of being Lean and Healthy for a Lifetime!

Our FYF4Good Power100 Heroes are AMAZING and so INSPIR-ING! This is why we call them "Heroes"! They are on a journey that will take them months or years and need all our love and attention. Some of them have tried twenty or more weight loss programs and are worse off for it. Some have had gastric bypass, sleeve, or balloon surgeries. Some have even done daily enemas to no avail. This breaks our hearts and our passion to help our obese Buddies runs very deep. We call them our Heroes because they are giving life another chance. We are 100 percent here for them. We know what FYF4Good can do to change their entire life with this *Lifestyle for a Lifetime!* Visit our website at FlushYourFat4Good.com to learn how to join the live support calls. We would love to have you on the call with us.

Archived Support Calls

Support calls, including the FYF4Good Power100 Heroes and selections from the original two test groups are recorded. There is an amazing support call library on FlushYourFat4Good.com where you will learn so much.

FlushYourFat4Good.com

This is the central hub where you can learn about and order the recommended supplements, request access to the Flush Your Fat 4Good "Buddies" Facebook Group, listen to archived support calls, find recipes, learn about the other books, enroll in the FYF4Good online courses, buy merchandise and so much more. Bookmark this website and use it frequently!

Flush Your Fat 4Good Online Courses

Visit FlushYourFat4Good.com for available online courses. At some point in your journey, you are going to want to learn more. When you feel you are ready, the courses are highly recommended for everyone living the FYF4Good Lifestyle. You will learn a lot about the science behind how FYF4Good works and you will personally benefit in your own journey by taking the time to take a course. Knowledge is Power. This valuable education will give you the confidence and information you need to embrace the FYF4Good Lifestyle and increase your chances for success for the rest of your life.

FYF4Good Buddies have the opportunity to take courses and learn at their own pace. The courses contain hours of in-depth training with Dr. Vicky and Jackie as they teach pearls of wisdom from sixty-plus combined years of hands on clinical practice and experience. You will not learn this anywhere else!

We also recommend that you schedule a session with one of our Senior Coaches! To get more information about personal coaching, visit FlushYourFat4Good.com. *"In order to win, you must participate."* —Jackie Padgette-Baird

Bring some Buddies with You

Who do you know that needs to lose some fat? Who do you know that needs to have more energy or sleep better? Who do you know that needs to feel better, have less aches and pains, more life in their day and more pep in their step? Who do you know that needs to be happier and in a better mood? Who do you know that is twenty pounds or more overfat and feels miserable with low energy, dragging themselves through life and struggling to move? Who do you know that is losing their quality of life, possibly having more frequent health episodes or prescribed more medications for conditions of aging? Perhaps diabetic medications, blood pressure medications, and diuretics for swollen ankles and fluid retention! Who do you know that has issues with their digestive system?

Bring them along on your journey! These people are all on a serious downhill path with their health. It is a matter of life and early death. Ask your friends and family to do this Lifestyle WITH you. They will feel better, and you will have an inner circle of friends and family on this journey!! This is about having good or better health, which is a truly important asset! The world can stop when good health is lost. FYF4Good can give you the tools and the control to help to take your health back!

Let's all get healthy together!

Get plugged-in on this Pillar! You need Support & Accountability to succeed, especially if you have a lot of fat to lose! WE ARE HERE FOR YOU!

CHAPTER THREE

FYF4GOOD LIFESTYLE PHASE I:

EATING AND NUTRIFYING TO LOSE THE FAT

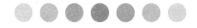

FYF4Good Phase 1 is designed to help you achieve an optimal healthy state of Accelerated Fat Burning. It is important to combine foods properly in their proper food groups, to carefully watch your digestion time, and to eliminate all starches and sugars (except for those coming from low-glycemic fruits and vegetables as they are naturally found in nature). By doing this, your body will be in Nutritional Ketosis and will start burning fat as your primary energy source. Your digestion will improve, and you will see many other health benefits.

FOOD COMBINING: DIGESTION TIMES OF FOOD GROUPS

You will need to pay attention to digestion times for each food group:

- Low-Glycemic Fruit: ALWAYS eat ALONE on an empty stomach, and after swallowing the last bite, **allow twenty minutes to digest**.
- FYF4Good Latte: This contains organic coffee with organic, unsweetened, plain, non-GMO recommended milk (soy, goat, hemp, or flax) and *FYF4Good Super Lean Aminos*. Eat when hun-

gry UNLESS the next food you are eating is fruit. In that situation, **allow one hour to digest** the protein in the milk before you eat the fruit. For optimal results, consume your FYF4Good Latte about thirty to sixty minutes before a main protein meal.

- Low-Glycemic Non-Starchy Vegetables: After swallowing the last bite, **allow two hours to digest.**
- Protein (animal, fish, fowl and plant): After swallowing the last bite, **allow four hours** to digest. **Pork, however, will take six hours**.

We recommend eating your protein with crunchy vegetables for two reasons: (1) Together they will slow assimilation and transition time through the digestive tract, keeping blood sugars level and sustained for the full four hours, and (2): Crunchy vegetables provide the fiber to "push" the poop through the gastrointestinal tract as well as "scrub" and clean the walls of the colon.

If you mis-combine, meaning you did not wait the proper amount of time to digest (e.g. eating fruit three hours after protein instead of four hours), it will take your body up to eight hours for your stomach to empty. During digestion, heat, acid and enzymes are released. Some foods require acid based digestive enzymes and some require alkaline based digestive enzymes. If both alkaline and acid enzymes are in the stomach together, they will neutralize each other, digestion will stop, and the food will start to putrefy, meaning it will start rotting inside you. This scenario can create gas, bloating, cramps, fatigue, and discomfort.

Extra Rule on Protein: Do not mix protein groups. If you are eating a plant protein (nuts, tofu, tempeh), only eat plant proteins. If you are eating flesh (animal, fish, fowl), stick with only flesh proteins. Avoid eating "Surf and Turf." This combination of proteins will bog down your digestive system and greatly slow digestion. It is recommended to eat water animals together and eat land animals together for better ease of digestion. For example: You can eat nuts on a vegetable salad, but you cannot eat nuts on Jackie's Chicken Salad because it has chicken in it.

Low-glycemic, non-starchy vegetables can be eaten with plant-based protein or flesh-based protein.

GOAT YOGURT FOR LONGEVITY

Goat yogurt is mandatory in FYF4Good. A common question is why can we eat goat yogurt (animal) and soaked nuts (plant) together? Great question! This is an amazing combination because both the yogurt and the soaked nuts are living organisms AND they contain enzymes, so they will digest beautifully. Also, you cannot "chew" your goat yogurt if you eat it by itself. By adding the soaked, live nuts to the goat yogurt, you can essentially chew the yogurt. This establishes better mastication in the mouth, where digestion starts, breaking it down to enter the stomach. The cultured properties of the yogurt allow for the nuts to be digested very well.

This is very interesting. Some of the longest living people are in Greece and are known to consume a tremendous amount of goat yogurt because of its probiotic benefits. FYF4Good recommends goat milk because it is the closest milk to human breast milk and is therefore so much easier to digest, especially for the elderly. The Island of Ikaria in Greece is one of the places on the list of the longest living populations. People on this island start their day off with goat milk and consume goat food products, including the meat. This leads one to believe that it could be of tremendous benefit to regularly eat goat yogurt. Yogurt provides good bacteria needed in the digestive tract. (By the way, the Ikarians also drink one to three cups of coffee a day.)

For variety, another great way to enjoy eating goat yogurt, instead of with nuts, chop up some cucumber, a little red onion, and add some dill weed into the yogurt for a delicious cucumber salad. Very tasty!

ELIMINATE STARCH IN PHASE I

It is CRUCIAL on Phase 1 to eliminate starches completely, including bread, potatoes, starchy vegetables, flour, and sugar. Eating starches, even just one serving, even a teeny, tiny bite of a piece of bread or cracker or cookie, will take you out of Nutritional Ketosis, the rapid Accelerated Fat Burning State (Pillar #1). It will take from one to four weeks to get back into full-blown Nutritional Ketosis—meaning one to four weeks before the body gets back to living off your stored fat for fuel. Just don't do it! It is not worth it. Be committed to getting your fat off … like yesterday … 4Good and get on with a new lean life!

By eliminating the extra sugar, starch, and starchy vegetables, your body will not be triggering insulin responses. Therefore, your blood sugar will stay at a more constant and consistent low level without a roller coaster effect. At this point you are burning stored fat, the premium fuel, instead of your carbohydrate rich food! Cravings for eating sugar and starches will miraculously disappear, and for most Buddies this is the most shocking experience of all. The loss of cravings will commonly occur within the first week or two. You will be amazed!

And one more comment on the timing of your food. Pillar #2: Food Combining (see chapter two) tells you how long to wait before you switch to a new food group. After swallowing the last bite of fruit, wait at least twenty minutes before switching to a different food group. After eating protein, wait four hours before switching to fruit. After eating vegetables, wait two hours before switching to the fruit. When eating protein, always eat vegetables (or nuts in the case of yogurt) with it to push the protein through the digestive tract. These are the minimum digestion times to wait to switch food groups. If you get hungry before the minimum time is up, you can stay within the same food group and eat something more. If you eat more protein, it will be four hours after you have eaten that new serving of protein before you can switch food groups. But remember; if you are hungry … eat. If you feel like eating protein, then eat it. Listen to your brain. Your body is dictating your needs to the brain.

FYF4Good does not recommend that you skip eating or wait too long before eating again. When you get up in the morning, DO NOT wait more than two hours before your first protein meal. That means that in your first two hours of the day, #1 eat a nice big serving of fruit, wait twenty minutes, #2 have your FYF4Good Latte, #3 then have a protein meal. Wait no more than two hours after you wake up to have that first protein meal.

Waiting too long is a common mistake when starting FYF4Good. The body needs protein early to rev-up the metabolism and get the fat burning. As you go through the day, DO NOT go more than five hours without food. Waiting too long causes blood sugars to drop and metabolism to slow. It is like throwing water on a burning campfire. You want that fire (metabolism) roaring. If you are hungry, we want you to eat! That will stoke the fire to burn the fat. We know this is not what you have been used to. However, along with training the brain, if you have a history of overeating or binging, your satiety center, the portion of your brain that signals the body when you are full, may not be working optimally.

We therefore recommend the following: When sitting down for a meal and you have eaten an average portion, but still feel hungry, relax and let your food digest by waiting at least ten minutes before taking a second portion. Allow your digestion to work and send the appropriate signals to the brain. For many, that pathway has been lost or even overlooked in the past because your eyes may have been bigger than your stomach, as the saying goes. This gives your body a chance to start listening for any signals coming from your brain, getting you more in-tune with your brain and satiety. If you are still hungry after waiting, then by all means eat more. *Do Not Overeat! Do Not Under-Eat!*

At the end of the day, you might need a snack before bed such as goat yogurt with nuts or a nice bowl of fruit such as cherries, or red grapes whatever fruit you have on hand. Eat it about one hour before bed. It is like having dessert! Do not go to bed on a full stomach, but alternatively do not go to bed on a totally empty stomach. If you do the later, your blood sugars could fall. You may wake up in the middle of the night and end up in your refrigerator!

MAKING SMART CHOICES

Buy fresh, organic, grass fed, local, non-GMO high-quality foods whenever possible. You want foods that are nutrient rich, absorbing as much nutrition as possible from your food and supplements. We live in a toxic world and the goal is to minimize the intake of harmful toxins: pesticides, herbicides, fungicides, and insecticides (see Pillar #5: Detoxing for more information).

There are a TON of foods for you to eat on Phase 1. Allow us to recap!

- Low-Glycemic Fruit: Refer to "Pillar #3: Low-Glycemic Eating" in chapter two or use the internet to search, "low-glycemic fruit" for ideas! Stay away from avocado and banana on Phase 1 even though they are low-glycemic. They slow down digestion because they are very dense and contain very little water. Stick with low-glycemic fruits that are hard to chew and are juicy. *The Harder to Chew, the More You Lose!*

- Low-Glycemic Non-Starchy Vegetables: Refer to "Selecting Fruits and Vegetables" in chapter eleven or use your internet search engine with "low-glycemic non-starchy vegetables" for ideas! Eat these raw or very lightly steamed or grilled. *The Harder to Chew, the More You Lose!*

- Cruciferous Vegetables: For the most part, these are best lightly steamed or slightly grilled with olive oil and seasonings, with the exception of Jackie's Chicken Salad where the raw broccoli florets are finely chopped, added to the salad and are digested well with the lemon mayo juice. Cruciferous vegetables such as broccoli, Brussels sprouts, and cauliflower when eaten raw can be difficult to digest, especially the stems as they can be fibrous. Other leafy cruciferous vegetables, including kale, cabbage, and arugula are great raw, but you may steam or lightly stir fry them as well. Be sure to remove the thick stems from the kale since they are woody and difficult to digest. In Phase 1, you want the impressive nutrients and cancer-preventive properties that cruciferous vegetables provide, which is why they are mandatory on FYF4Good. Once the beneficial nutrients are recognized and brought into the cells, the nutrition will speed up the mitochondria or power house of the cell and start the process for burning fat. If this is new for you, your Buddies will be there to help guide you and help you to learn how to identify them and prepare them properly.

- Protein: chicken, turkey, eggs, seeds, nuts, fish (fresh, local, wild, non-toxic), red meat (grass fed), pork (six hours digestion time for pork), for vegans and vegetarians choose tofu, tempeh, and nuts and seeds.

- Nuts and Seeds: These are to be raw and then soaked overnight with Pink Himalayan Salt, rinsed and dried on low heat in the oven or dehydrator.
- Dip for raw vegetables: Use organic, unsweetened, non-GMO, EDTA-free mayonnaise with a squeeze of lemon (Jackie's Lemon Mayo Dip) or soft goat cheese. Keep in mind, if you choose goat cheese, it is a protein food not a fat. It will take longer to digest than the Jackie's Lemon Mayo Dip. Protein digests in four hours.
- Yogurt: Use organic, unsweetened and plain goat, sheep, or soy yogurt (soy for vegans and vegetarians only) with a handful of soaked nuts or seeds. You may make your own yogurt, but do not use rice, oat, or cow milk.

More About Taking Nutritional Supplements
It is Essential to Nutrify
In our discussion of Pillar #4 we talk about which supplements are highly recommended. The FYF4Good website has a list of where you will find these supplements to satisfy the requirements of Pillar #4: Nutrifying. Please refer to both our book and our website, contact your Buddy or Coach for more information, ask questions in the Facebook Group or jump on a live weekly support call. Pick your supplements wisely and make sure you have what you need. Human cells must be supported to perform all their functions.

Important Instructions for Taking Supplements:
- Probiotics are taken right before your head hits the pillow at night. Should it be necessary to take the recommended Colon Health supplement, take *one hour* before you take your probiotics.
- Digestive enzymes are taken ten to twenty minutes before every protein meal. Make it a habit to take them as you are preparing your meal. (But if you forget to take them before your protein meal, take it as soon as you remember, during or after the meal, even if an hour later.)
- *FYF4Good Latte: Super Lean Aminos (Muscle Building-Fat Burning Powder)* is mixed with organic coffee and recommended milk. You always drink this first thing in the morning, at least twenty

minutes after your low-glycemic fruit. And again later in the day after your second serving of low-glycemic fruit. You may have a third FYF4Good Latte (with or without the coffee) if you wish.

- Core supplements are taken twice a day. Once in the morning before or after your fruit and once in the evening before or after your fruit. Take these with your CranFlush.

- And do not forget to be drinking the minimum recommended amount of CranFlush, eighty-one ounces, everyday!

There is a reason for everything we do and everything we eat with the FYF4Good Lifestyle. It has been shown that the recommendations of the FYF4Good Lifestyle, when followed to a "T," results in safe rapid fat loss, plus an abundance of energy due to the maximum absorption of nutrients.

A TYPICAL DAY ON PHASE 1: LOSING THE FAT

Give your body the very best start each morning. After sleeping seven to eight hours, you will be eating on an empty stomach. Your probiotics have been populating all night long, just waiting for your fruit to come down. Not only is the fruit great food for those little guys but they have been waiting to extract the nutrients from your food. They transport the nutrients to the walls of the small intestine. Next the villi hairs and mucosa cells help deliver the nutrients into the bloodstream to feed all parts of your body. Cool huh? The human body is just absolutely amazing!

BREAKFAST! Breaking your Fast!
Low-Glycemic Fruit
- First thing in the morning *run* to have a big serving of low-glycemic fruit and take your supplements with your CranFlush. When you finish your last bite of fruit, take note of the time. Wait at least twenty minutes. Use the time to mix your CranFlush needed for the day and to make your first FYF4Good Latte. No almond or coconut milk. These milks have very little if any protein content, so they are not to be used for your FYF4Good Latte. For fun and

great taste, get a frother or a whisk to foam up your FYF4Good Latte. If made correctly, this latte will have approximately twenty grams of protein. Enjoy lots of cinnamon and/or a dash of cayenne pepper on top to add spice. It is also a thermogenic!

FYF4Good Latte

- Twenty minutes after swallowing your last bite of fruit, drink your FYF4Good Latte!

Protein and Vegetable Meal

When hungry, usually thirty to sixty minutes later, you will be ready for a protein and vegetable meal. This should be eaten within two hours of waking up.

- Take your digestive enzyme supplement before your protein meal! If you happen to forget, take it as soon as you remember, during the meal or after.
- IMPORTANT: do not drink liquids while eating your foods because they will dilute your digestive enzymes reducing your ability to optimally digest!!
- CHEW your food thoroughly, at least thirty-three chews per bite. There should be very little to swallow if you have chewed correctly.
- Ideas for your protein meal:

    Eggs cooked any way you want: hard-boiled, soft-boiled, scrambled or in an omelet. Add vegetables (asparagus, broccoli, kale, spinach, onions, mushrooms), fresh salsa, goat or sheep cheese to make Jackie's Three-Egg Omelet! If you are vegan, eat tempeh, tofu, soy cheese. You might also try Jackie's Egg and Veggie Muffins. (Refer to chapter nine: "FYF4GOOD Staples" or visit FlushYourFat4Good.com for the recipe.)

    Chicken, turkey, or "clean wild" fish (NEVER farm-raised) with vegetables or in a salad.

    Jackie's Chicken Salad (refer to chapter nine: "FYF4GOOD Staples" for the recipe). You can make this with chicken, turkey, eggs, or fish (tuna or salmon are great!) Tempeh, tofu, Spice of Life Meatless Meats ONLY if vegan. BE CREATIVE!

Raw vegetables with Jackie's Lemon Mayo Dip.

Goat or sheep yogurt, soy yogurts for vegetarians and vegans, with a handful of soaked nuts and/or seeds.

CranFlush

Drink CranFlush All Day Long!...but when you are eating meals, do not drink any liquids. This is very important, as it dilutes your digestive enzymes, making digestion less efficient! You can drink right before your meals to eliminate thirst during your meals. If you are thirsty during your meal, as well as right after the meal, take only a couple of small sips. About one hour after you have completed the meal you can resume drinking your CranFlush or any other liquids.

Mid-Day

- If it has been four hours since you finished your first protein meal, this would be a great time to have your second serving of low-glycemic fruit! However, you might want more vegetables or protein. Listen to your body! If vegetables or protein sound good to you, and you are really hungry, then wait until evening to have your second serving of fruit.
- Take the recommended digestive enzymes! Try NOT to forget as this really helps with fat loss.
- Mid-Day Meal ideas include:

  Any of the protein ideas previously mentioned are also great here!

  A large vegetable salad (arugula, kale, peppers, cucumbers, onion, celery, zucchini, etc.) with Organic, Unsweetened, non-GMO, EDTA-free Mayonnaise with a squeeze of lemon. Add your favorite lean protein.

  Grilled fish and grilled asparagus with Jackie's Crispy Garlic Brussels Sprouts.

  Turkey burger, no bun, wrapped in lettuce with tomato and a little goat cheese.

Sardines with a little onion, squeeze of lemon, and sliced red bell peppers.

More goat or sheep yogurt with nuts/seeds.

The options are endless.

Eat until you are full! Listen to your brain, that inner feeling or voice. Remember, FYF4Good *Trains Your Brain!*

CranFlush

Remember to drink CranFlush all afternoon! You must get at least eighty-one ounces in by the end of the day!

Mid-Afternoon

- If you find your stomach growling, this is a great time to just grab some raw or slightly grilled, low-glycemic, non-starchy vegetables. Remember it takes two hours to digest these.

Late Afternoon / Dinner

- If you have not had the second serving of low-glycemic fruit, now is the time to do it! But make sure it has been at least four hours since your last protein meal and at least two hours since your last vegetable meal.
- Take your second half of your daily core supplements with your CranFlush.
- After twenty minutes of fruit digestion, it is time to have your second FYF4Good Latte.
- Take your digestive enzymes ten to twenty minutes before you start eating your protein and vegetable meal!

CranFlush

Continue to drink CranFlush throughout the evening!

We make CranFlush in an 800 ml Voss bottle. Mix one-part unsweetened, not from concentrate, 100 percent cranberry juice with four or five parts filtered water. For the CranGingerFlush, add a teaspoon to a tablespoon of freshly juiced ginger root to the CranFlush.

We use the large glass Voss bottle for several important reasons. It is made from glass, not plastic, so we know we are not getting any of the chemicals that can be leached out of some plastics. It has a good size mouth, which promotes drinking more liquid. We can wash the bottle with a long bottle brush and use it over and over again. It is a very large bottle and when you have it sitting around you, you will be compelled to drink from it. Additionally, if we are all drinking from the same bottle, when we talk on the support calls or Facebook, and someone asks, "How much CranFlush did you have today?" we know that everyone is talking about the same thing.

Later Evening

If you have not had your second serving of fruit, it is important to eat it before you go to bed. Also, if you have not had goat yogurt with soaked nuts during the day, the evening is a great time to enjoy a bowl of it! Many Buddies on the Lifestyle find this to be a nice dessert to end the day. Sometimes they place it in the freezer for a while before eating it for a thicker texture.

Before bed, take your probiotic, brush your teeth and get at least seven to eight hours of restful sleep before starting your next day.

The Pattern

Repeat day one on day two and on day three and day four and on your remaining days in Phase 1. Keeping in mind that *You Can Never Go Wrong Eating Right!*

Keep your days very simple when starting Phase 1. Do not get carried away with your recipes. Simple is better when retraining the brain.

Have Jackie's Chicken Salad at least once a day, every day for the first three months! Think we are kidding? Not at all! Jackie's Chicken Salad was completely designed to play a major role with fat loss. There was a method to Jackie's madness! Chicken is relatively easier to digest than other heavier proteins. Chicken is packed with nutrients, especially the branched chain amino acid leucine, helping you to burn fat and build lean muscle mass. The more lean muscle mass you have, the more you will lose.

Muscle burns fat. All the other ingredients were intentional to perpetuate rapid fat loss. You will love it, your body will love it, and it will accelerate your fat loss! All the Buddies tell us their spouses and kids love it too. So make it for the whole family.

Stay the course, and trust the process! If you make some mistake or mess up for example by getting the timing wrong, do not be so hard on yourself or beat yourself up. There is a learning curve with this Lifestyle. Continue to move forward and focus on your goals from meal-to-meal. Look ahead to the next food that you will be eating. As long as you do not eat the forbidden starches and sugars, you will most likely remain in Nutritional Ketosis even if you make a mistake in Phase 1.

Stay on Phase 1 until you know you have lost ALL of your excess fat and you like how you look when standing in front of the mirror naked. It is up to you, and not the scale! Do not make your decision based on the scale weight. The scale is a liar and will not tell you the truth. In fact, throw it away because you do not need it! You will be creating lean muscle mass and possibly building bone density. Muscle weighs more than fat. This is what you truly want for your heart. And the lean muscle also makes you shapely.

That is all you need to know for FYF4Good Phase 1!

But what about calories, portion control, egg whites only, white meat vs dark meat, not eating after 7:00 p.m.? … DON'T WORRY ABOUT IT! As we said in the beginning, *all that you thought it was, it's NOT!* Believe it or not, FYF4Good really does not have a lot of rules. It might be very different for you to understand the digestive timings, but you will come to find this Lifestyle is really very easy.

DO NOT OVEREAT! DO NOT UNDER-EAT!

When you are hungry your brain is telling you that you need to eat, so eat! On this Lifestyle you are going to be eating yourself lean. Within a very short time, you will know when it is time to eat because you will become in tune with when your stomach has emptied. You will be able to tell time by your digestion! We do not want you to ever be really hungry or "starving." Your body will hold onto your fat or create more for a survival mechanism. Your brain will decide, and you will get the message. *FYF4Good Trains Your Brain!*

CHAPTER FOUR

FYF4GOOD LIFESTYLE PHASE 2:

EATING AND NUTRIFYING

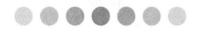

A Lifestyle for a Lifetime!

Once you have lost all your unwanted fat, you are ready to start Phase 2 of *A Lifestyle for a Lifetime!* It is up to you. YOU are in complete control now. Huge congratulations for the journey you have taken to this point.

Phase 2 is not for the next sixty, ninety, or one hundred twenty days. It is for the rest of your life. Your body is on the road to the best health it has been in, maybe in your entire life. This will continue, provided you stay true to Phase 2. Do not slip back into filling your body with sugars and toxins. Continue to properly combine your foods at all times. Eat healthy foods, nutrify, and continue to flush. Your choices will determine your destiny.

For those of you that have just lost twenty, fifty, eighty, one hundred or more pounds, not only have you drastically reduced your chances of premature death, but you have also reduced your risk for at least twenty health conditions.

FYF4Good is not temporary. It is a way to live long, to not suffer, and to improve your health. It is a way to enjoy the fruits of your labor and feel amazing while you journey through life. This is a great journey!

ADDING STARCHES IN PHASE 2

For Phase 2, starches will be introduced back into your Lifestyle. If you find you are starting to get out of control with the starches, as sometimes that can happen, go back to Phase 1, and stay on it for at least two weeks before you introduce starches again. It is easy to go back on Phase 1; it is always there for you and should be second nature. You have control and can take charge of the situation by eating according to Phase 1. This is why we recommend that you should always follow Phase 1 when traveling. If you found you mis-combined and need to get back on track, or if you really are not enjoying the way starches make your body feel, Phase 1 baby, FYF4Good is the blueprint for optimal health. You are in the driver's seat and now have the knowledge and power *to Be Lean and Healthy for Life!* We want you to be your own guru with this amazing knowledge.

In Phase 2 it is advised to not have more than one meal containing starch during a day. Please understand that you do not need to have a starch meal every day (or any day for that matter). In fact, many of our Buddies prefer to alternate two to three (or more) days on Phase 1 and then one to two days on Phase 2. You get to decide, as your brain will tell you if it is a Phase 1 day or a Phase 2 day. But just as when you are on Phase 1, you need to plan. So if you know you are going to have a starch meal later in the day, do not have starch in the morning and vice versa! That could be overkill for you. Some of our Buddies decide that they want to feel as fantastic as they did while on Phase 1, so they choose to stick more to Phase 1. If you have a birthday or a Mexican restaurant night out and you want those tortilla chips, guacamole, and salsa, then do Phase 2 that day. You call the shots!

Remember: Sugar Stops Digestion. **SUGAR STOPS DIGESTION**! So if you really, really, want that piece of birthday cake or special dessert, do NOT eat it after a protein meal. It is best to have the dessert on a completely empty stomach to provide the best chance to get it through your body quickly. After eating the dessert, wait two hours before switching food groups. Double up on your digestive enzymes before eating it, and then go right back onto Phase 1 eating for several days. If you are going to eat the dessert right after your meal, for example the cake on your birthday, make the meal a starch meal. NEVER eat sugar two days in a row! You will regret it if you do, so do not do it! Remember, sugar acts like cocaine on the brain.

The 8 Essential Pillars still apply for Phase 2. With all the toxicity in our world, toxic exposure is inevitable every day. You need to continue to Detox (Pillar #5) and Flush (Pillar #6). You do not have to drink as much of the CranFlush every day, but most of us do. You might also notice that you still drop inches in some areas of your body, even while you are on Phase 2! Your body will continue to drop until it has reached the best body composition. Your brain knows best!

In Phase 2 your digestion times are the same as Phase 1. We are still food combining now and forever! By now you know your food groups and how long digestion takes for each. You are adding starch in Phase 2, which is what is different. Here is a quick review:

- Low-Glycemic Fruit: After swallowing the last bite, allow twenty minutes to digest.
- Avocado, bananas, or high-glycemic fruit (above sixty glycemic index): **Allow thirty minutes to digest.**
- FYF4Good Latte: Drink your latte and then eat your next food when hungry UNLESS the next thing you are eating is fruit. If so, allow one hour to digest the protein in the soy milk and two hours for goat milk before eating the fruit. *The FYF4Good Latte is optional in Phase 2, but most of us cannot give it up since it is so healthy and has so many great benefits.*
- Low-glycemic non-starchy vegetables, starchy vegetables, other starches: After swallowing the last bite, allow two hours to digest.
- Protein: After swallowing the last bite, allow four hours to digest (pork takes six hours to digest).

We still recommend eating protein with crunchy vegetables in Phase 2. This is important for your bowels. Remember: If you mis-combine, meaning you did not wait the proper amount of time to digest, it will take your body eight hours to get back on track! So make your choices wisely! Otherwise you will feel bloated and uncomfortable. Who wants that, and what is the point?

Morning meals are a great place to start introducing starches back into your Lifestyle. Take this slow and easy until you get the hang of it.

If you have a tendency to retain a lot of fat, it is recommended that you continue the FYF4Good Latte in Phase 2. From clinical experience, we have seen it can take up to two years for your body to adapt, readjust, and stabilize. You have completely changed your body composition, and the body will continue to improve, so commit to the Lifestyle 4Good. We recommend staying on all the supplements, especially while the body is stabilizing. Your heart is a different size, blood vessels that are not needed are dissolving, and your entire body is adapting. This could mean there is a lot of healing and cleansing going on, as well as muscle and bone growth. The cells need to be fed properly by nutrifying to perform all their functions. Try to stay the course with your supplements. If you have a financial challenge, connect with us via the support channels for recommendations on what you can do to nutrify during Phase 2 and continue the Lifestyle. Remember, you only have one body, so do the very best you can!

Believe it or not, many people that do not have any fat to lose, love doing Phase 2 just for health reasons. People who are not well typically choose to do Phase 1 and then go to Phase 2 as the health conditions improve. Sugar and starches can increase the severity of a health condition, so this is why many people stay on Phase 1 during the duration of their condition. Remember this is all about digestion, absorption, and elimination.

A Phase 2 Day Is Exactly Like a Phase 1 Day Except for Adding the Starch Meal

- Fruit, then CranFlush (recommended but not mandatory in Phase 2) with supplements. Wait twenty to thirty minutes depending on if it is low-glycemic or high-glycemic fruit.
- Organic coffee with recommended milk, or take it black if you like. However, having it with milk is better on your stomach and provides extra protein. If you have your FYF4Good Latte *(optional in Phase 2),* wait thirty minutes if you are having a protein meal or

one hour if you are having more fruit. If you are using goat milk in your coffee and having a starch meal, wait at least two hours.

- Starch Morning Meal Introduction

    First Week: After your fruit (and waiting twenty to thirty minutes), one to two slices of Ezekiel or any organic, unsweetened sprouted bread, lightly toasted with organic and/or raw butter. Consuming the starch with a fat is a must as it lowers the glycemic index. Avocado is great to eat for the fat, too. After a starch you will now wait two hours before another food group.

    Second Week: Now you can eat your sprouted bread with organic butter or organic RAW nut butters. Make sure your nut butters are fresh and raw (not roasted), especially peanut butters. Also, you can add healthy sprouted grain cereals. NOTE: "plant" milks combine with grains. Goat milk does not combine with the grains. Ezekiel tortillas are great with mayonnaise spread all over, sprinkled with Pink Himalayan Salt, a little cayenne, and then add vegetables like asparagus, broccoli, red bell peppers, sprouts, avocado slices, kale and arugula, and squeeze a little lemon all over. Roll up for a great veggie roll. (Use Press'n Seal by Glad, Saran wrap or aluminum foil to hold it together.) Enjoy baked sweet potatoes with butter or coconut oil.

    Third Week: Now that your body has become accustomed to the reintroduction of starches in your Lifestyle, you are in pretty good shape! Enjoy your healthy sprouted grain cereals and sprouted bread with your butter, ghee, raw nut butters, avocado, veggie rolls and sweet potatoes.

    Fourth Week and Beyond: Now you have got decisions to make! You can have a "starch" meal if you choose, or save your starch meal for later in the day. If saving it for later in the day, have protein and vegetables for your meals earlier in the day.

- The rest of the day is the SAME AS PHASE 1 (for the timing of supplements, CranFlush, and food combining).

Examples of Great Starch, Grain, Legume, and Starchy Vegetable Ideas

- Organic non-GMO quinoa, amaranth, steel oats, and/or millet (avoid "quick" one-minute or microwave oats or grain products): Soak overnight in water with one tablespoon lemon juice and one tablespoon Pink Himalayan Salt. When ready to eat, drain and rinse, add water, and cook. Add organic butter or coconut oil.
- Ezekiel Bread with avocado, arugula, kale, romaine lettuce, sprouts, squeeze of lemon, sea salt, and cayenne pepper.
- Sweet potato with butter, coconut oil or olive oil (baked or steamed). *Hold the marshmallows.*
- Salad with vegetables, grilled eggplant, and Ezekiel tortillas. Add salsa and guacamole!
- Beans and rice—No white rice since it is polished. Use organic long-grain brown rice or basmati rice instead. Soak the beans in water overnight before you cook them. Change the water several times. It will bubble up because the protein is digesting the starch. Soaking overnight can cause the germination and release of the enzymes as well. When you eat beans, you get gas because it is a protein and starch mis-combine if the beans have not been soaked. Do not eat animal and fish proteins with beans. You can eat plant proteins with beans. Also rice and beans together make a complete plant protein.

Examples of Good Meal Choices
Italian Food
- Pastas, salads, breads
- Meats and Vegetables
- DO NOT eat protein and pasta together! It is a mis-combine.

Sushi
- California roll without crab (be aware that the rice, unless it is brown rice, may have sugar mixed in it to make it sticky). Do your research on your restaurant's quality.
- Tempura vegetables, but not with shrimp

- Seaweed hand rolls with fish and lots of vegetables, no rice
- Sashimi with salads (e.g. cucumber salad), but no rice
- Teriyaki chicken or beef, vegetables, cucumber salad

Mexican

- Find sprouted grain tortillas for homemade food
- Healthy rice and beans with avocado or guacamole, salsa, chips, salad
- Rice and bean tacos, no cheese or meats
- Pinto or black beans, guacamole and salsa roll into a burrito with a tortilla
- Chicken, fish, meat with vegetables, salads
- Tostadas with meat, vegetables, guacamole, and salsa—do not eat tortilla shell
- Chicken, beef or fish fajitas, but with no tortillas or rice and lots of vegetables and salad, salsa, guacamole

Soups

- Jackie's Turkey Soup with greens and vegetables only. No rice, grains, beans, pasta or bread.
- Chicken with vegetables (no rice, macaroni, pasta, or noodles)
- Vegetable broth / vegetable soup with rice, macaroni, beans, or grains
- Cream soups must not have starch in them unless soy or goat milk is the cream. Keep in mind soy is a plant protein. Therefore, grains are ok in your vegetable soup. Goat milk will be ok with your chicken, turkey or beef soups.
- Beef stews with vegetables and no potatoes

Other

- Zucchini boats with beans, vegan cheese, tomatoes, sprouts, red bell peppers, avocado, and onions
- Chicken with vegetables (no rice, macaroni, pasta, or noodles)
- Spaghetti squash mixed with eggs and baked with vegetables and goat/sheep cheese and no starches

- More recipes are on FlushYourFat4Good.com and in the Flush Your Fat 4Good "Buddies" Facebook Group

Mis-Combined Meal Examples
- Proteins with starches
- Chicken and rice
- Meat and potatoes
- Bread and meats
- Fish and rice
- Eggs and toast or eggs with hash browns
- Spaghetti and meatballs
- Pancakes and sausage
- Tortilla and meats

Alcohol

We do not drink alcohol in Phase 1. We are giving the liver a break; we are detoxing and flushing. The liver is a fascinating and complex organ. It is said that it has one million functions. A healthy liver is critical for us to be healthy.

Alcohol ingested goes straight to sugar and into the bloodstream. It is absorbed in the digestive tract and metabolized in the liver. Perhaps you have heard that alcoholics can be suffering from liver disease. If you drink too much alcohol in one sitting, some liver cells will die and be replaced by fat (steatosis). This occurs in 90 percent of people who drink too much alcohol.

Another function of the liver is to metabolize the fat and help to remove toxins from the body.

Additionally, one of the main functions of the liver is to detoxify the colon, large intestines, or bowels. So, during Phase 1, we eliminate alcohol to give the liver a break to work hard for rapid fat loss, detoxing, and flushing.

If you choose to drink alcohol, in Phase 2, here are some rules for doing that:
- Consume the alcohol on an empty stomach. This will prevent it from being poured onto your foods, which will mess with your digestion. Also, it will mean that you will need less alcohol to feel the effects, so you will consume less and, good news, pay less!

- If you are going to have a meal with your alcohol, a starch meal is best. Finish your drink, and then eat. Starch will absorb the alcohol and help to process it.
- If you are eating protein and vegetables, finish your drink. Then eat your vegetables first, and then eat your protein.
- We recommend you do not drink alcohol every day. Save it for special occasions.

Other Uses for Phase 2

- **Pregnant women or nursing mothers**: FYF4Good highly recommends pregnant or lactating women seek advice from their primary physician before starting this Lifestyle. The nutrients received from the starches can be beneficial in pregnancy. Therefore, from decades of clinical practice, Phase 2 has been demonstrated to be GREAT during pregnancy. We have already had our first FYF4Good baby that was born to a mom who lost a significant amount of fat on Phase 1, then moved on to Phase 2 and was on Phase 2 during her entire pregnancy. Mom and baby are doing fine and EXTRA BONUS.... Mom returned to her pre-pregnancy (post Phase 1) weight VERY quickly! The extra fat just melted away! Remember, you are what SHE ate. Preparing to have a baby (or currently pregnant) and eating the FYF4Good way is a great benefit for a great outcome.
- **People who really do not have any fat to lose**, but they want to be healthier. Phase 2 will help take the burden off digestion, returning digestion to optimal working order, leading to better health. We all can benefit from eating this way! You will not get too thin. Fat will be shed if the body determines it. We cannot see the visceral fat surrounding and crowding out our organs and it cannot be removed by liposuction. The benefit will be better digestion, absorption and elimination. Remember, the digestive tract comprises 70 to 80 percent of the immune system! So healthier digestion will help anyone's immune system.
- **People who need to gain weight!** Yes, there are a few of them out there. If you feel like you are too thin, and you want to gain

weight, it is important to do it in a healthy way! In many cases, digestion is not optimal, and there is poor absorption leaving the person deficient in nutrients. It is certainly okay to follow Phase 1 for two weeks and then move on to Phase 2. No one is going to get too thin on Phase 1. Phase 1 and Phase 2 will aid in digestion and help absorption for optimal health. It will help to put on lean muscle mass, and still keep body fat at a minimum.

Eating anything you can get your hands on, especially "junk food," to gain weight would not be a good idea. It is our view that junk food does so much damage that it is not safe to eat, not even once! Talk about giving the liver a work out! Eating unhealthy foods containing starches, sugar, and iodized salt can lead to unhealthy cells that are functioning at less than optimal levels. We are only as healthy as our cells. All diseases start in the cells. Ultimately, eating unhealthy foods can also lead to excess visceral fat. You may not see it, but your body will begin to show signs of it as your well-being and function diminishes. And you certainly will not gain bone and muscle, which is essential for optimal health.

Instead of guessing what you should be eating, follow FYF-4Good Phase 2. One tweak to make to the plan if you want to gain weight, is to drink your FYF4Good Latte thirty minutes AFTER your meal instead of thirty minutes before your meal. This drink is designed to add additional protein to your Lifestyle and help build lean muscle mass because there are branched chain amino acids. They are designed to keep or build lean muscle mass while burning stored fat. Drinking the FYF4Good Latte before the meal triggers the satiety center in the brain and therefore curbs the appetite. This makes it so effective in Phase 1. Taken after meals in Phase 2, you will continue to build more lean muscle mass instead of focusing on burning the fat. Regardless of whether you are in Phase 1 or Phase 2, if you mis–combine foods by choice or by accident, do NOT do this two days in a row.

Remember: *Do Not Overeat! Do Not Under-Eat!*

ADVICE FOR VEGANS AND VEGETARIANS

The FYF4Good Lifestyle is terrific for vegetarians, vegans. lacto-ovo-vegetarians, and pescetarians (pesco vegetarians). It is easy for vegetarians and vegans to become overfat, because starch is often part of every meal. Yeast overgrowth is common. Muscle mass suffers in this group, as well. Regardless of your eating style, most people do not eat enough protein every day. In FYF4Good Phase 1 there are no starchy vegetables, grains, cow dairy, sugars, sweeteners, artificial sweeteners, or dyes allowed. To do this right for a vegan or vegetarian, protein is the name of the game!

- **Vegans:** Follow the instructions for Phase 1. (Refer to chapter three, "Phase 1: Eating and Nutrifying to Lose the Fat.") However, you will substitute the meatless meats and tempeh for the animal meats that are suggested. You may also consume soy, hemp, or flax milk; soy, hemp, or flax yogurt; hemp hearts; soaked raw nuts and seeds; tofu; and soy meatless meats (no sugar added).
- **Vegetarians:** Consume the same as vegans, but you may also have goat milk, goat or sheep cheese, and goat or sheep yogurt. NO COW DAIRY in any form.
- **Lacto-Ovo-Vegetarians:** Consume the same as vegetarians, but also include eggs.
- **Pescetarians (Pesco Vegetarians):** Consume the same as lacto-ovo-vegetarians, but also include fish. We do not recommend shellfish because they are bottom feeders and their livers contain neurotoxins. Consume only wild fish, never "farm-raised," which can be very toxic.

A great source to find healthy meatless meat is Spice of Life Meatless Meats! Ground-round, chicken, and beef chunks are all good choices. Avoid the jerky because it has sugar.

Use these meatless meats, eggs, or fish to make the recipes in the book and on FlushYourFat4Good.com. You can use the chicken pieces specified for Jackie's Chicken Salad or substitute the chicken with fish or eggs. You can also make a Tofu Scramble with lots of vegetables and cut up soy sausage (with no sugar) and soy cheeses. Bragg Liquid Aminos is acceptable for your seasoning as well. Use recommended milks only in your FYF4Good Latte two times per day. Organic coffee is mandatory, and you may drink up to three cups per day.

Basic Phase 1
- Eat soy, hemp, or flax unsweetened yogurt with soaked nuts or seeds every day.
- Take your supplements with your CranFlush as directed.
- Remember not to eat any starchy foods in Phase 1 until you have reached your goal size and go into Phase 2. Do not eat legumes such as beans or hummus. No grains, noodles, rice, bread, or any starchy vegetables, including potatoes, yams, sweet potatoes, corn, cooked carrots, etc. Use your internet search engine for a complete list of starchy vegetables to avoid.
- Your goal is to consume mostly proteins and non-starchy vegetables during your day. Follow this *Lifestyle to a "T"* and you will have great results!
- There are close to twenty grams of protein in your FYF4Good Latte with the recommended milk and *FYF4Good Super Lean Aminos (Muscle Building-Fat Burning Powder)* that will help you to accomplish building your lean muscle mass and have rapid fat loss.
- Eat low-glycemic fruits at least twice a day.
- Consume CranFlush (at least eighty-one ounces per day).

Important Note:
Vegetarians, Lacto-Ovo-Vegetarians and Pescetarians: Eating your plant protein (tofu, tempeh, meatless meats) with your animal protein (goat milk, goat or sheep yogurt, goat or sheep cheese, eggs or fish), is *mis-combining*!

- Digestion time of goat yogurt with nuts is four hours.
- If you have a salad with goat or sheep cheese, make a large vegetable salad, and wait four hours for digestion.

- If you eat eggs and fish, you may mix the goat or sheep cheese with it. Wait four hours after eating to switch and have your tofu, tempeh, meatless meats, or fruit **because technically the plant proteins are somewhat starchy.**

When you reach your ideal weight, and you like how you look in the mirror, NAKED!, you may go to Phase 2. FYF4Good will teach you how to eat by incorporating your grains and maintaining your weight for the rest of your life without ever struggling again.

CHAPTER FIVE

TRAVELING, SPECIAL GROCERY
SHOPPING, EATING OUT, AND HOLIDAYS

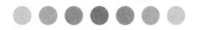

Remember the 5 P's ... Proper Planning Prevents Poor Performance!

TIPS FOR TRAVELING

The key to success when traveling is to plan ahead. By planning, you will succeed. Regardless of whether you are on Phase 1 or on Phase 2, it is always best and so much easier to eat Phase 1 foods while traveling. You will reduce the risk of mis-combining foods, and it is easier to order in restaurants. You may think it will be difficult, but it is not! You are in control, remember that. FYF4Good Buddies consistently report they come back from traveling three to five pounds lighter or their clothes fit looser!

Whether you are traveling by car, boat, plane, train, bicycle, or hiking, you will feel better if you plan in advance and stick to it. Remember, this is *A Lifestyle for a Lifetime!* Your health is an important asset! Maintaining good health needs to be taken very seriously, and you will be glad you did.

If traveling by car, you may have more flexibility because of the extra space, and everything is easier to transport. That being said: Apply these tips to your mode of transportation, when possible.

Car Trips
- Make sure to have a BIG COOLER (or two) stocked with your favorite Phase 1 meals and snacks to keep you satisfied. Each day you can add more fresh ice to keep everything cool. Ideas include:

Ziplock Bags with fresh, grilled or chopped vegetables: asparagus, broccoli, carrot sticks, celery, peppers, cucumbers, cherry tomatoes, and zucchini. Bring a little Tupperware of Jackie's Lemon Mayo Dip for veggies. Remember, *The Harder to Chew, The More You Lose!*

Fruit: apples, pears, strawberries, blueberries—whatever is in season and low-glycemic. Fresh is always best!

Have a bottle (or two) of unsweetened, not from concentrate, 100 percent cranberry juice always cooling down. Lemons to squeeze in your water, especially if you run out of your cranberry juice. Ginger juice is great with the lemon juice as well.

Pre-steamed artichokes with Jackie's Lemon Mayo Dip in a little Tupperware container

Single-serving containers of Jackie's Chicken Salad

Precooked turkey or beef meatballs

Hard-boiled eggs

Precooked stuffed bell peppers made with ground turkey, chicken, lamb, or beef

Soft goat cheese (for vegetable dipping)

Yogurt: organic, unsweetened, plain goat or sheep (soy for vegans and vegetarians)

Soaked nuts and seeds: pecans, walnuts, pumpkin, sunflower seeds: have them ready to go.

Organic mustard

Organic, unsweetened, non-GMO, EDTA-free mayonnaise

Goat milk or goat milk powder

Soy milk or soy milk powder

- Pack enough jars of your unsweetened, not from concentrate, 100 percent cranberry juice and your organic, unsweetened, plain, non-GMO recommended milk (soy, goat, hemp or flax) to last the entire trip. It can be left in the car and ready to go when you need a new container.
- Bottled purified waters to keep hydrated and to prepare Cran-Flush

- Plastic silverware, napkins, paper plates, cups, Ziplock bags, glass water bottles
- Ground organic coffee, a frother (If you do not have room for the frother, a whisk or two plastic forks held with the points facing away from each other works great) and a water heater for the hotel room to make your coffee if the hotel does not have a coffee maker.
- Bring a fine-meshed small wire strainer or a small French press for a single cup of coffee.
- Your supplements! Make sure you take enough for the entire trip!
- Extra Ziplock bags are your best friend.

Check FlushYourFat4Good.com for nifty containers and ideas for traveling.

Air Travel

When traveling by plane, train, or boat, pack in a double Ziplock bag two to three boxes of your soy milk in your luggage along with your ground coffee and soaked nuts. You can even pack goat yogurt in your luggage, double bagged, but not sealed airtight so that the air pressure change does not pop open the container. This gives some immediate options when you arrive at your destination.

For the plane, take as many three-ounce plastic bottles filled with unsweetened, not from concentrate, 100 percent cranberry juice as allowed in your carry-on. Freezing them the night before is always a great idea to keep them fresh. Once through security, buy one or two large bottles of water and immediately make your CranFlush. You of course will have packed a lot of food (see ideas in the previous section) in your carry-on. It is difficult to find healthy food options at airports and impossible once you board the plane. You never know when there might be a delay, plane re-routing, or cancellation, even with very short flights.

When traveling, never ever, ever, allow yourself to get hungry and not have food. This just sets you up for a mad dash to find an option that may only result in an unhealthy choice and many times a choice that could throw you out of Nutritional Ketosis and make you feel sick.

Remember *The 5 P's—*
Proper Planning Prevents Poor Performance!
And man, does it!

TIPS FOR GROCERY SHOPPING

Whether in your hometown or traveling abroad, if you run out of food, or just need some new options, use your internet search engine to find the nearest Whole Foods, Trader Joe's, or Sprouts. Also try putting "Health Food" or "Healthy Foods" into your GPS. You will be surprised at the number of suggestions that pop up!

Most grocery stores now have whole rotisserie chickens, hot food bars, and/or salad bars. Try to always stay ORGANIC or GRASS-FED when selecting your meats, butters, and other food.

Always stock up on lemons to squeeze in your water for extra detoxing. While traveling abroad, the correct type of cranberry juice is difficult or impossible to find. But lemons or limes are usually available.

When you traverse the grocery store, stay on the outside isles, those close to the walls. This is where you typically find your fresh fruits and vegetables, goat yogurt and cheese, meats and poultry, as well as pre-cooked foods and salad bars. You may need to venture down an aisle or two to find the right type of soy milk (you should be able to find an option that can be stored on the pantry shelf—probably in the cereal aisle), powdered soy milk, cranberry juice, or nuts. But for the most part, what you need is all around the edges of the store. If goat milk is hard to find in your travels, then get the proper soy, hemp, or flax. Hemp or flax can be difficult to find. So those on goat milk, get the powdered goat milk for the duration of your travels. You can also get powdered soy, unsweetened as well.

Always remember to BUY FRESH when you can. Do not buy frozen fruits, vegetables, and meats, etc. Additionally do not buy fresh produce and freeze them if you have other options. The process of freezing and thawing breaks down the properties of the food and denatures them. If it is difficult to find fresh foods in your area, flash-frozen fruit and vegetables are better than canned. And many times they are picked ripe, which means they have matured and contain phytochemicals, cancer prevention micronutrients.

FOR HEAVEN'S SAKE, READ THE LABEL!

"I have been saying this for years. *'If God made it, EAT IT. If man made it, READ IT.'* Most of the time if you read it, you are throwing it out!" —Jackie Padgette-Baird

Our modern society has become accustomed to eating processed, pre-packaged, and fast food items. Although these choices may be convenient, they are far from healthy options. Some experts even refer to them as "edible food-like substances." In FYF4Good, we do not consider them to be edible! PERIOD! Here is why . . .

The foods around the perimeter of the grocery store are, for the most part, fresh, natural foods occurring in nature. These items are placed on the perimeter because they need to be restocked often, as they do not have a long shelf life. These items include fruits, vegetables, fresh meats, and dairy items. This is where you will find most of the items that we eat on FYF4Good!

The items located in the center aisles of the store have a very LONG shelf life. That is because they are processed and contain high levels of pre-servatives and other chemicals. These preservatives and chemicals are not good for the human body. For optimal health, STOP eating prepackaged foods that contain high levels of salt (sodium), preservatives, chemicals, food colorings, added sugar, artificial sugars, and bad fats.

So what should I be looking for on the label?

Stay away from these:

- The chemical EDTA—this is used as a preservative, often found in mayonnaise and other foods.
- High-fructose corn syrup—First of all, most of the corn and corn derivatives in the food chain are GMO. Second, this is made in a chemistry lab. It contains poisonous chemicals. As you begin to read more and more labels, you will notice that high-fructose corn syrup is in MANY boxed, bagged, and canned items in the grocery store. When you see it on the label, put it back on the shelf and walk away.

- Artificial food colorings should not be consumed.
- Sugars or sweeteners added, such as high fructose corn syrup, malto-dextrin, dextrose, sucrose, fructose, maltose, erythritol, Stevia, etc.
- Partially hydrogenated oils (trans fats)

Synthetic nutritional products should also not be consumed. At best, the human body does not absorb or recognize the synthetic product, so it will become toxic and stored in fat cells or eliminated immediately by the body. At worst, synthetic nutrients cause major health issues. Several studies designed to prove that synthetic nutrients were safe had to be halted because diseases and the mortality rate of the group receiving synthetic nutrition went up compared to the group not getting it. (See studies discussed in *New England Journal of Medicine* in 1995 and 1996.)

Synthetic vitamins build up in adipose tissue (fat). As fat is shed by the body it is processed by the liver, resulting in a congested liver.

Synthetic nutrition comes in the form of supplements, but it also comes in the form of additives to prepackaged food. It is a cheap, chemical substitute for real nutrition. It is cheap because it is made from coal tar, petroleum, petroleum by-products, ground-up rocks, iron shavings and/or chemicals, which the human body is not designed to digest. It is added to prepackaged foods (including baby foods) to give them the appearance of being healthier, but they are NOT healthier. They can also make you deficient in other important vitamins and minerals. So they do more harm than good.

Look for US Pharmaceutical (USP) Grade supplements on the label and any ingredient ending in the suffixes "-acid," "-ide," "-ate" or that use "dl" before the name. These vitamins are man-made in a lab. Also, another clue is sugars, syrups, and fractionated oils that might also be on the label. This will tell you these vitamins are not of the best quality and should not be added to your Lifestyle.

TIPS FOR EATING OUT

When eating in restaurants, remember to ask for the food to be prepared exactly the way you want it. Be specific! You are paying for it!

Ask for sauces and dressings on the side, and ask to substitute grilled or steamed vegetables or sliced tomatoes for the usual potatoes or toast. Ask for lemon and olive oil or lemon and mayonnaise for your salad dressing. Always ask them to remove the bread basket or stack of crackers from the table. If fruit comes with your meal, ask for a "to go" container, and have it later in the day or the next morning.

When ordering an omelet a couple of things to ask are:

- Do they use real eggs? (No egg substitutes.)
- Do they add milk or pancake batter when making an omelet or scrambled eggs? It is true; pancake batter is added to egg omelets in many restaurants. Tell them you must have only real, fresh eggs.
- If you want cheese in your omelet, it must be cheese from GOATS or SHEEP. If they do not have either one, leave out the cheese!
- Have them fill the omelet with crunchy vegetables like peppers, kale, spinach, broccoli, or asparagus, and ask for fresh salsa. Remember, *The Harder to Chew, the More You Lose!*

Do not stress out. This is easy to follow, and most restaurants are ready to accommodate special requests (especially when you tell them this is about your health). The more they accommodate you, the more you will return to their restaurant. And do not forget to bring your soy, goat, hemp, or flax milk and your supplements to the restaurant if you need them! Should you find in your food any breading, cooked tomatoes, or anything else not allowed on Phase 1, such as croutons in your salad, just scrape them off or remove them.

BUT WHAT ABOUT HOLIDAYS OR DINNER AT A FRIEND'S HOUSE?

Remember *The 5 P's... Proper Planning Prevents Poor Performance!* Think about eating something before you go so you are not famished when you arrive. Having a bowl of goat yogurt with nuts or a serving of Jackie's Chicken Salad will allow your body to think less about what to eat and more about connecting and enjoying the other people you are with. Eating a big serving of fruit and drinking a FYF4Good Latte before going is another idea to keep your appetite at a minimum. And, of course, take your

CranFlush with you! If you are going to a potluck event, take something with you that you can eat. This guarantees you have options.

When it is time to fill your plate, double up on the protein—roasted turkey, chicken, prime ribs—as well as all of those roasted vegetables and dressing-free salads. Do not put anything on your plate that is not allowed in Phase 1. Do not ever allow yourself to be "guilt-ed" into having "just one bite" of grandma's mash potatoes or Aunt Emma's chocolate cake. It is always best to tell the truth. You are focused on improving your health and have given up sugar and certain starches. Or if you think they will truly be insulted if you do not have some, tell them you would like to take it "to go" so you can enjoy it later. Make sure it is given to a friend or tossed out before you arrive home. Do whatever you need to do to keep it out of your mouth and house. In many cases, this is life or death. That is how serious we take this Lifestyle since we have watched, as you may have as well, the demise of loved ones due to obesity or poor choices of food.

No need to hurt yourself with bad food to have a good time!
— Jackie Padgette-Baird

You are in control!
Do not allow anyone to derail your progress 4good!

CHAPTER SIX

GLOBESITY

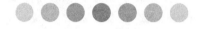

Obesity is now all over the globe!

The definition of "obesity" is the condition of being grossly fat or over-weight. According to the World Health Organization, worldwide obesity rates have more than doubled since 1980.

Globesity refers to the global nature of the obesity problem. Globesity is not just a problem in Western nations, and malnutrition is not just a problem in third-world countries. Severely underweight and overweight people are BOTH suffering from malnutrition as neither body condition properly absorbs nutrition. The modern-day diet is killing people and many just turn their backs and want to blame people for over or under eating. They do not look at why they are eating this way.

Obesity is responsible for three hundred thousand (300,000) deaths every year in the United States alone. The United States is now the leading country in rate of obesity (percentage of the population that is obese) according to the *Obesity Update 2017*, by the OECD (Organization for Economic Co-operation and Development). This is shocking!

As early as the mid-1800s, "fatness" has been measured by calculating the body mass index (BMI): the ratio of height to weight. Although this measurement has been used in the past, and is often considered accurate, it is not a good indicator of fatness at all! Here is why: Two people both of the same height and weight will have the same BMI. But if one is an athlete in top condition and has a lot of lean muscle, and the other never exercises, eats poorly, and has very little lean muscle, well you can see where BMI is misleading.

Research, like that published in the *International Journal of Obesity,* showing alternatives to BMI can be easily found: body adiposity index, waist circumference, waist-to-hip ratio, hydrostatic weighing, air displacement plethysmography, body-fat measuring, bioelectrical impedance scale, and dual energy X-ray absorptiometry, to name some of them. A DEXA scan is currently one of the most accurate ways to measure your fat, muscles, and bones. The test can be costly but will give you one of the best readings of your overall body composition.

FYF4Good uses inches or clothing sizes to measure progress instead of weight or BMI. Stay off the scale! Do not be a scale-aholic. Instead, break out a standard sewing tape measure (can be purchased in drugstores, hardware stores, and where sewing supplies are sold) and track your progress. Know that the scale lies to you! On FYF4Good, you begin to build lean muscle mass and bone density, so if you think you lost ten pounds you might have really lost twelve pounds of fat and gained two pounds of bone and muscle. The only accurate test would be to have a DEXA scan.

THE CONSEQUENCES OF BEING OVERWEIGHT AND OVERFAT

While we do not like to admit it, most people know if they are overweight. The hard-cold truth is if you carry twenty or more excess pounds of fat on your body you are dangerously overfat. Here are some interesting facts:

- An overweight person with elevated cholesterol is guaranteed to see those levels fall if they return to normal weight.
- Overweight Americans that are age twenty to seventy-five have 1.5 times greater risk of having higher cholesterol.
- Younger people are at the greater risk of having higher cholesterol. Overweight Americans, age twenty to forty-five, have a 2.1 times greater risk than older adults.
- Every 1 percent decrease in cholesterol results in a 2 percent decrease in the risk for heart disease.

- Eighty percent (80 percent) of diabetics are obese.
- Type 2 diabetes, although considered a mature disease, will not manifest until obesity sets in.
- If you are obese, you have a higher risk of heart disease, stroke, diabetes, dementia, and cancer, and the list goes on and on.
- As a consequence of globesity, the global presence of NAFLD (Nonalcoholic Fatty Liver Disease) is 24 percent.
- Quality of life is reduced when a person is twenty pounds (or more) overfat.
- It is more likely for obese people to develop arthritis in their weight bearing joints (knee, ankle, and spine). "Arthro" is a prefix meaning joint. "-itis" is the suffix that means inflammation. When there is too much weight on a joint, the bones are pushed closer together. As the joint space narrows it becomes irritated. Inflammation sets in. This sends a signal to the brain that there is a problem in the joint and it needs to stop moving. The body develops bone spurs, tiny pointed outgrowth of bone, which develops into osteoarthritis. This can occur in an area of injury or inflammation of the local tendons or cartilage. The body will try to "bridge" the joint with spurring to stop movement and further damage or inflammation. The good news is that once excess weight is taken off, the bone spurs *can* reabsorb.
- A man weighing twice his ideal weight has a twelve times greater risk of dying from accidents than a man at his ideal weight. Why? An overfat person loses track of where their body is in space, their reaction time is slowed, their body is too heavy to control, joint mobility is limited and, in general, men take more risk and perform more dangerous physical work.

Just twenty pounds of excess fat increases the chances for developing a multitude of serious health conditions. The following are some of the many health conditions caused by being overfat:

- diabetes
- cancer

- congestive heart failure
- enlarged heart
- pulmonary embolism
- polycystic ovarian syndrome
- gastro-esophageal reflux disease
- fatty liver disease (Nonalcoholic Fatty Liver Disease)
- hernia
- erectile dysfunction
- urinary incontinence
- chronic renal failure
- lymph edema
- cellulitis
- stroke
- pickwickian (obesity hypoventilation) syndrome
- depression
- osteoarthritis
- gout
- gallbladder disease

If you look at the skin of people who are dramatically obese, it looks like it is going to burst. It is tight and puffy. Extra water is being stored in the tissues below the skin. This is an unhealthy storage of water and indicates that the body is not functioning correctly. This will reverse and return to healthy functioning through the FYF4Good Lifestyle.

WHY DO PEOPLE BECOME OVERFAT?

There are many contributing factors to the reasons a person becomes overfat: caloric intake is too high (emotional overeating); eating foods with no nutritional value and high calories (junk foods); lack of exercise; sedentary jobs or sitting too much; insulin resistance; diabetes; many medications may cause the body to retain excess liquids or increase the production of fat; a thyroid not working correctly (hormone imbalance); genetics; eating the wrong TYPES of foods such as too many starches and sugars; decreased metabolism due to age; postpartum hormonal imbalance; female menopause; male menopause; stress; psycho-emotional reasons (i.e. emotional binge-eating) and always hungry, and therefore eating constantly because the nutrients the body requires for functioning are not present in the low-quality foods being eaten. Combinations of these, as well as many other factors, are reasons people become overfat.

What many overfat people have in common is they have lost control of their endocrine system. The endocrine system includes eight glands in the body, one of which is the master gland, the pituitary gland in the brain, which sends the messages to the other glands to balance the hormones in the body. But in overfat people the hormones become chaotic. As one hormone gets out of balance, the endocrine system tries to correct and rebalance, but cannot. The effects cascade, and the system will not function properly, eventually causing real health issues related to multiple hormonal imbalances. One of the most common hormonal health issue is thyroid imbalances. Being overfat can typically cause depression, a feeling of hopelessness, lack of sleep, and fatigue.

Here is one of the mechanisms to become overfat. When the body needs insulin to control sugar spikes, the pancreas secretes the hormone insulin into the blood stream. Eating starches and sugars trigger the brain to command the pancreas to secrete insulin. Eating exclusively or too many of the starches and sugars will cause spikes and surges of insulin or an insulin response. This creates sugar in the bloodstream and will cause the body to make fat. When the body is seriously overfat, the pancreas secretes too much insulin into the blood stream. This leads to sodium and water retention, improper metabolism of sugars, and a body that is unable to utilize its stored fatty acids.

Additionally, the body cannot utilize insulin properly, so it will continue to make more insulin. Blood sugar is elevated despite overproduction of insulin in the blood because the cells are not responding to insulin (insulin resistance). Because of the overload of insulin, eventually a mechanism is turned on where the body may completely turn off production of insulin altogether as a result of this state of insulin resistance and the condition of prediabetes.

The state of insulin resistance in the body will ultimately reduce the level of neurotransmitters in the brain, most importantly serotonin. Proper serotonin levels are needed in the body for mind well-being (good feelings) and for good quality sleep. Lowered levels cause depression which is unfortunately, very common in obesity. Consuming starches and sugars is really the "slow poison" perpetuating this cycle of insulin resistance and lowered serotonin levels.

What happens to the body if you eliminate complex carbohydrates, starches, sugars, and high-glycemic fruits and vegetables (anything that would instigate an insulin response)? A landmark study from 1985 published in the *American Journal of Public Health,* included obese subjects with obesity related problems including: borderline diabetes (pre-diabetes), hypertension, elevated blood pressure, elevated cholesterol, trouble walking, pain in the knees, fatigue, low energy, depression, and sleeping problems. Measurements were documented at the beginning of the study and again at the end of the study. The results were game changing. All problems—everything—improved and the subjects started losing weight. Vitamin and mineral supplementation was required along with counseling and support, and when the target goal was achieved, a maintenance program was started adding carbohydrates gradually.

CHAPTER SEVEN

FYF4GOOD POWER100 HEROES

GLOBESITY DOES NOT HAVE TO BE

You have finally found what you are looking for! I know because I have seen this work for hundreds of people. Just like YOU! Just like ME!

I was in denial when I found FYF4Good. I knew I had a lot of weight to lose (about one hundred pounds), but when I looked in the mirror, I saw myself thinner than I really was. After I lost about sixty pounds, I started to realize just how bad I had allowed things to get. I also knew that there were some hurts from my past, as well as some patterns of thinking and living, that allowed me to get that big. I knew that if I didn't make some changes in my thoughts, feelings, and decisions, I would probably gain the weight back after reaching my goal. And if that was true for me, it was probably true for some of the other FYF4Good Buddies as well.

People with a lot of fat to lose have struggles, issues, and questions that someone with five or ten pounds to lose just won't understand. The most common question that I am asked is, 'What about your skin? Did it shrink or is it flabby? People with five pounds to lose don't even think to ask that question.

So, I asked Dr. Vicky and Jackie for a forum where Buddies with a lot of fat to lose (fifty, one hundred, one hundred fifty, two hundred plus pounds) could interact with each other and encourage each other in hope and healing. And thus was born the FYF4Good Power100 Heroes, a special group of courageous individuals who are now a team. We are a grass-roots initiative to shift the paradigm of the way people see the fat loss journey, and we are making a tremendous impact! If you are significantly overfat, do not wait one more day, we would love to have you join us!

~ Coach Jennifer, FYF4Good Power100
Heroes Host Lead and Buddy

Meet Our Power100 Heroes

First of all: IT IS NOT YOUR FAULT! It is not your fault that you got this big. Look around you. We are an obese society. *Globesity*, which is defined as obesity seen as a global social problem, is here. If you go to an event or a function such as a graduation, wedding, baseball game, football game, or amusement park, take notice of how many people are twenty to thirty pounds or more overfat. Most likely it will be at least half of the people. Globesity is all around you. It is pandemic!

Because of the way many of the foods we eat are grown and processed, they lack adequate nutrition and give little opportunity for the average person to be healthy. Coupled with our crazy, busy, rat-race lifestyle, we have little time to take the effort to prepare a really healthy meal. It is so much easier and more convenient to pick up some fast food or what we call "junk food." Often we hear about easy to prepare frozen or fast food from our friends or family and what is advertised on TV, radio, in magazines or on billboards, which influences us to try them.

Information remains limited about the "real" nutritional value of food. The nutritional content of the foods we are eating, whether they are good or bad and how they affect our health, is not taught well in schools. People want to trust that they are being told correctly how to maintain a healthy lifestyle. But this is often not the case. Take for example the government in the 1980s telling us to follow their famous food pyramid. People listened to this advice for at least a decade. At the top were all grains, starches, starchy vegetables, and low-fat foods. This is how you fatten cows. Cows are supposed to eat grass not grains. This is why 80 percent of our population is low in CLA (Conjugated Linoleic Acid). CLA is an essential fatty acid that prevents the enlargement of fat cells, breaks them up and builds lean muscle mass; plus provides an array of major health benefits.

With easy access to the internet and many books and articles available on the subjects of good nutrition and cooking healthy food, the trend is that more and more people are educating themselves about how to eat well. Because there are so many diet suggestions out there, and a large number of these are not healthy, it can be very confusing. FYF4Good is based on biochemistry and physiology, it is easy to understand and it is easy to know why it works.

On the other hand, many people remain stuck in the paradigms passed down from our parents, grandparents, and other relatives about how they think about their food—what to eat, when to eat, and how much to eat. "Clean your plate or you cannot have dessert!" Many of us have traditional cultural foods (healthy and unhealthy) that we were raised with. We eat food when we are sad or angry or happy (comfort/emotional eating). As a result of all of this pouring into our conscious mind, our subconscious mind has developed and imprinted a paradigm that keeps us where we are because of the relationship we have with our food. And eventually, it often makes us sick and fat.

When you eat foods low in nutritional value, your body is not getting enough nutrients, so it signals you to be hungry. Thus you eat more. People keep eating and eating because the brain is signaling the body that nutrition is needed. Snack foods and junk food are "empty," hefty calories loaded with sugars and bad fats. As we overeat to try to satisfy the body's needs, the pounds of fat slowly creep on. It is so gradual that we do not realize it is happening. A person who is one hundred or more pounds over-fat is malnourished—period—and they are essentially ill. A starving child in a society that is food-deprived is emaciated and likewise malnourished. There is no difference between the two individuals from a core-health perspective.

The cycle is about to be broken!

You are not alone on this journey. Thousands of people have successfully walked this path before you. The FYF4Good Lifestyle works, and there are so many healthy, happy, lean people to prove that it does.

Do not wait even one more day to start. Did you know that just twenty pounds of extra fat puts you at an increased risk of over twenty serious health conditions? Your family needs you. Your friends need you. And you need to fulfil your purpose here on Earth. You need to take care of this NOW!

And what about how you FEEL? You may not think you are depressed, but chances are very good that you are. It is a physiological fact that your hormones are in chaos. You may be the life of the party and can joke around to distract yourself from the pain, but deep down inside, ask yourself if you are truly happy. When you get up in the morning are you excited about life, and are you looking forward to the day ahead? Probably not. It might be difficult or painful, maybe even impossible just to get out of bed, let alone move around. "Emotional eating" can contribute to gaining extra fat as one eats food to try to find "comfort." Many of us have used food to numb our pain. If this sounds like you, you are not alone. Depression, exhaustion, exasperation, hopelessness, sleeplessness, and brain fog are all very common in overfat individuals. The sad thing is that doctors will give drugs for these symptoms before they talk to their patients about their diet.

But here is the good news: As you eat in a safe and healthy way to lose the fat and change the composition of your body, all this will change. Your hormones will begin to balance out. You will come out of a brain fog that you may not have even recognized. Your joints will not hurt as much anymore. You will have more energy to do the things that you need and want to do. You will sleep more deeply and wake refreshed. Your blood testing and other lab results will start to look better. YOU WILL BECOME A NICER PERSON! And you will become HAPPIER. Seriously!

In the FYF4Good Power100 Heroes community, we will help you work through these issues and more. We are here for you and we cannot wait to follow your success. We are thrilled because we know that if you follow this *Lifestyle to a "T"* you will never struggle again, and it will only get better and better for you.

Here are some things to do to get ready for your journey:

- First, clear your home completely of all temptations. Get your spouse and your family that you live with to help you. This means candy, ice cream, chips, crackers, cereals, breads, etc., need to GO! Wherever something not permitted is hiding—in the pantry, the refrigerator, the freezer, under the bed, in the closet, or in the garage—give it to neighbors, friends, or a food pantry. Better yet, throw it out.

You may say, "Oh, I will just stick the M&Ms in the freezer for the grandkids." No! Get it out of the house! It is poison to your body and to theirs. Would you let them get into a box of pesticides? No, of course not! So why give them this poison?

There will be times when you might feel weak or get tempted. You do not want anything close by that will derail your progress and commitment to your life. You are going to be re-programming your brain on this journey. It is going to take some time, but do not worry, it will not take forever. So, do not tempt yourself during the process.

- Ask those around you—your family, your friends, and your coworkers—for support. Share with them that you are making a change in your life for your health. Ask them to support you in this change. If they need to get healthy, ask them to Buddy-up with you so that you can support each other. This means that instead of going out for Friday night pizza, you will go to a place with more healthy choices or enjoy cooking at home.

One of the biggest challenges you will face as you lose the fat is the reaction of the people closest to you. At first, they are going to be skeptical of FYF4Good. Maybe they have seen you try lots of other things in the past. Early on, some of them might try to talk you out of starting this because they think you are going to fail again, and they do not want you to be hurt. Again! Not the best support!

- Not everyone will be supportive of your decision. Some may be envious of your transition. Yes, you heard right. People will feel happy for your success, but they might feel miserable because of deep feelings of hopelessness, wishing they could do the same. And there are some people who only feel good when they have someone else close-by who is in worse shape than they are, not because they are mean or hurtful people, but because it empowers them. They want to keep you right where you are in the "misery loves company" club with them. When you start getting lean and healthy, they are going to realize that you are doing what they have failed so many times to do, or what they do not have the discipline or the courage to do. Hopefully that will encourage them to make a Paradigm Shift for the better, like you did.

People generally do not like any kind of change; they will try to sabotage your success to keep you where you were. This is a selfish attitude. It is done out of fear and not to purposely hurt anyone. They just do not want you to change because they think they may lose you. The best thing to stay on track is to avoid these people until you are strong and confident enough to share with them what you have been doing. Then you can encourage them to take up this healthy Lifestyle for themselves. But for now, nothing is more important than your health, and if they cannot support you, it is best to limit your time with them, or completely detach from them.

This is one of the most important reasons why we have the 8th Pillar and the FYF4Good Buddy system, which includes Coaches, support calls and our Facebook Group. Reach out to receive support and accountability from your Buddy and/or Coach. Talk about this and ask them to help keep you strong to stay the course. Nothing is more important than your health. Having good health is your most important asset, and if family, friends, and relatives cannot support you, limit your time with them for now. It is also a possibility that they will push you away in their fear and/or jealousy. If this happens, know that it is not your fault. Stay the course no matter what! Reach out to your FYF4Good Buddies and they will help you through this adjustment.

- As you begin this Lifestyle, take several "before" pictures and your measurements. You never have to share any of this with anyone else, but they will be important points of reference for you to measure your success. You will not be able to fully understand your journey without the pictures. Here are some tips for your "before" pictures.

Take your pictures in soft lighting that will not cast awkward shadows across your face or body.

Find a spot with a neutral background with little distractions behind you. A blank wall or a door makes a good background.

Wear clothing that contrasts in color with your background. If the wall is light colored, wear dark clothing. If the wall is dark, wear light clothing. Do not blend in with your background.

Try to wear form-fitting clothing or even your bathing suit. These pictures are for you, but hopefully, one day you might want to share them with your Buddies. Your success might help just one other person.

Take several pictures at different angles. Face the camera, face away from the camera, face right, and face left.

Of course, this means that a friend will need to be working the camera for you (unless you have a tripod and a timer).

Consider saving this outfit to use for after pictures. Some Buddies have put back on the same outfit and it makes a very striking picture as the outfit becomes baggy.

Store your pictures in at least three places, your computer and two backup flash drives, so that they do not get destroyed. Consider saving them in "the cloud" or on Facebook so that they are remote from your home, just in case.

- Record your "before" weight and your measurements on the measurement chart in the Flush Your Fat 4Good Workbook (available to print out on FlushYourFat4Good.com). After that, DO NOT step on the scale for at least thirty days. The scale is a liar. In fact, THROW AWAY THE SCALE! As you shed the fat 4Good, you will be gaining lean muscle and bone. The scale is not an accurate account of your progress. Your measurements, clothing sizes, and changes in how your clothes fit, will be more accurate.

On this journey, the scale is taboo. For those of you scale-aholics who feel compelled to get on it daily, or even several times a day, DON'T DO IT! Your weight will fluctuate throughout the day as you eat, drink, and eliminate. This is not reflecting your fat loss. Let the way that you feel and the way your clothes fit be your motivation on your journey. You will have a special kind of freedom when you no longer own a scale.

- If you are like most of us, you probably have numerous sizes of clothes in your closet and many in dark colors. When you have a little extra time, organize your closet with the largest sizes in the front, the smallest sizes in the back. As you are on this journey, you will be dropping clothing sizes rapidly. Some people drop one or two sizes a month!

    As a size gets too big for you, box it up and donate it. Get it out of the house. You will no longer go back to those clothes, ever again, in your life!

    Others of us got rid of the smaller sizes as we lost hope in ever getting smaller again. If that is you, check out thrift stores in your area for the in-between sizes as you lose pounds. You do not want to pay department-store prices for clothes that will fit for about a month. There are many thrift store options in most cities, and you can find brand new clothes with the department store tags still on them or find used clothes that look like they were never worn, at ridiculously low prices. These stores often have sale days as well. Ask when their next sale will be. This is a terrific idea because on FYF-4Good there will be rapid fat loss. You may only be able to wear that smaller size pant, shirt, or top for a couple weeks. Buying second hand clothes will be cost effective until you reach your goal size.

- Early in your journey, make it your habit to get on the LIVE support calls, especially the FYF4Good Power100 Heroes Call. Coaches who have dropped about one hundred pounds host this weekly call. Dr. Vicky and Jackie are usually on the call for questions and support. This is where you can hear what other people are going through, ask questions, share your results, and be inspired! You can put your phone on "mute" and go about your business as you are listening in. Some people listen while they are making dinner! It is a huge help to be on the call. You might hear just one thing that catapults you into next week with excitement. We hear this from our Buddies all the time. If you miss a call, recorded calls can be accessed on FlushYourFat4Good.com.

- Remember, the 5 P's: *Proper Planning Prevents Poor Performance!* Always prepare your food and supplements the night before. This sets you up for success. We call it "Habitual Ritual." This helps to establish better discipline too. If you are running late, or just need to eat something healthy because your blood sugar has dropped, having multiple individual servings of Jackie's Chicken Salad pre-made, goat yogurt with nuts, or Jackie's Egg and Veggie Muffins ready to go, will help. Tupperware will be your best friend. Goat yogurt with nuts is great for a fast get away. Clean and cut up raw vegetables and make some Jackie's Lemon Mayo Dip. Have your fruit already cleaned and packaged in sandwich bags. Get on the FYF4Good website and our Facebook Group for more ideas on food to go! *You Can Never Go Wrong Eating Right!* Try to get really good at being prepared! It will accelerate your results and you will feel really great about being in control.

- No matter how busy you are, get your thirty minutes of exercise at least five days a week. There were studies done in several countries regarding the absolute most effective and healthiest exercise routine. Walking is the best for losing fat. Exercise will accelerate your progress and promote better health. If you physically cannot walk for thirty minutes, or if you have walking restrictions, do what you can, and each day try to add a tiny bit more. Do exercises in bed if you are bedbound. Add ankle and wrist weights as you do them. The muscles burn your fat. Build them up. If you are a woman, you will not get bulky because you do not have as much testosterone as a man. You MUST get your body active and moving to achieve optimal health. Read "Pillar #7: Exercise & Sleep" in chapter two for more ideas.

- It is critical, critical, critical that you have at least eighty-one ounces of CranFlush every day. It is more critical for you than a person who is battling to lose ten pounds of fat. Why? Because you will be burning a LOT of fat, and that fat is full of toxins. You will be burning it so fast that your liver can become congested with the fat and toxins. Your kidneys will be overwhelmed as well with filtering the blood. You want the toxins out of your body as fast as you can get them out. And you want to take the burden off the liver by taking in lots of fluid to flush the fat. The CranFlush is excellent for flushing toxins and fat out of the liver and kidneys and keeping them clean!

- CAUTION! When you are in a grocery store, stay on the perimeter. Never walk by candy, sugar, ice cream, crackers, chips, and cereal. You do not want to trigger your brain to crave these items. Eventually you will no longer be tempted, but in the beginning, this is very critical. If you feel weak, immediately call or text your Buddy with a "MAY DAY! MAY DAY!" and they will help you through it. Just try to keep in mind that those foods are abusive, and you no longer will accept being abused.

- If you are at a point where you start craving sugar, immediately eat some protein. Make sure you are drinking your CranFlush and are hydrated as well. Do not give in to birthday cake or other holiday eating. The holidays will come around again next year. One little bite of sugar or flour will take you out of Nutritional Ketosis. If you get your body out of Nutritional Ketosis, it can take your body from one to four weeks to get back into full-blown Nutritional Ketosis, rapidly burning fat for fuel. UP TO FOUR WEEKS! JUST DON'T GIVE IN! You have worked too hard up to this point to blow it on a bite of cake! That sets your journey back up to four weeks. During that time you could be down another six to ten pounds of fat. If you were able to trade six pounds (or more) of fat off of your body for not eating a piece of cake, would you do it? You bet you would ... and that is exactly the choice you will be making!

No need to hurt yourself with bad food to have a good time.
— Jackie Padgette-Baird

- Whenever celebrating birthdays or other special occasions, make sure that there are options for you to enjoy, like a huge bowl of berries, vegetables stuffed with ground turkey and yummy goat cheese, or a big bowl of goat yogurt with nuts. It is very important to ALWAYS combine your foods correctly! Make it a point to cement this into your Lifestyle so you do not get yourself into trouble.

- If you make a choice to eat sugar, your brain will be triggered, thinking that it is a reward or a treat, but really it is not. It is poison. *Sugar is like cocaine on the brain!* It is a drug. It will set you up to go back down that road you were on. Save the sugar until all the fat is off your body and make the decision at that time. At that point you will decide, "Do I want to have this food in my life once or twice a year?" But not now! Wait until you are on Phase 2, you will be able to eat certain treats at the proper time and be in control and stay lean and healthy. We will teach you how. Some of what you think you might want, when you get to Phase 2, you will not even think about or want.

- Never, ever, ever skip a meal. If you are hungry, eat. Do not think that by skipping that meal you will lose fat faster. This is a new paradigm. You will not be counting calories on this journey. Many of you are afraid to eat for fear that you will gain weight if you do. That is the old paradigm. You know the rules of eating now, especially food combining, and you are in complete control. Before, chances are pretty good that you did not practice food combining. So, yes, eating more and not combining your foods properly, will put added pounds on the body. In this Lifestyle, eating will not do that. *Do Not Overeat! Do Not Under-Eat!* If you are hungry you MUST EAT. If you are not so hungry, just eat a little bit, but EAT! *It Stokes the Fire to Burn the Fat!* If you stick with the old paradigm and starve yourself, this will slow down the fat burning process, because now your body will go into conserve mode. Your metabolism will dramatically slow down and nothing may happen in your fat loss. Shift your paradigm and eat; throw kindling on the fire to keep the fire (metabolism) going and the fat burning. If you ever went camping and the fire burned low, you put more twigs and branches on the fire to keep you warm all night. Right? The same is true for our bodies. For more information, read the section on "Why Diets Don't Work" in the introduction chapter.

- When you have reached your three-month anniversary of clean Phase 1 eating, take new photos and record your measurements. Pull out your original photos and look at them side-by-side with the new pictures. Post your new picture on your refrigerator or your bathroom mirror as the new you. This is very important to Re-Train Your Brain to see the new, healthier, smaller you! The choice is yours. Be happy and grateful that you have made the shift to change your paradigm *to Be Lean and Healthy for Life*. Write it down and say it at least three times a day to yourself. "I am so happy and grateful that I have made the commitment to change my paradigm to *Be Lean and Healthy for Life!*" You have no idea how powerful it will be to hear yourself say those words and truly feel what you are saying. By truly **feeling** these words, you will start **thinking** thoughts in a different way and your thoughts will create your **new reality**. You will be amazed at how lean and healthy you will become by just feeling true gratitude and appreciation of the body God has given you and the power you now have over it.

Congratulations on your decision to start this exciting journey. This WILL work for you as long as you work the 8 Essential Pillars and follow this *Lifestyle to a "T"* carefully.

And remember, you are not alone; your Buddies are here for you every step of the way!

CHAPTER EIGHT

REDEFINING YOUR SELF-IMAGE

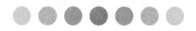

You are what you think you are!
Time to put on a new pair of glasses!

WHAT GOT YOU HERE?

Learning, and following to a "T" the FYF4Good 8 Essential Pillars is critical for you to rapidly achieve a body that is not only lean, but one that is in optimal health. It is all based on biochemistry, which is real nutrition. Science and decades of research support the main features of the 8 Essential Pillars and the benefits to living the FYF4Good Lifestyle. The physical transformation you will be making, especially if you are currently carrying a lot of extra fat, will be life changing! If you are on the road to losing fifty, a hundred, two-hundred pounds or more of fat, the "new you" will be transformative!

But just as important as the physical transformation, you must experience a mental (and often emotional) transformation—and this one may be a little harder. Why? It is different for each of us. What might work for one person, may not for another. There are so many factors that have affected not only how we look at and value our own self-worth, but why and how we became overfat. The mental transformation is necessary to ensure that the physical transformation does not reverse.

The truth is that even though you might be shrinking, for many people, your conscious mind (your thinking mind) is still convinced you are fat. We call this "Distorted Body Awareness" or DBA. Your brain may still perceive that you are bigger than your actual size. Carrying lots of fat for a long time can create distorted perceptions and can become the dominate brain image, rising into the consciousness. This could explicitly affect the way a person views their body. Short-term fat gain and then loss is an acute situation. However, being overfat for a long time changes your self-image, and that DBA becomes a permanent image in your brain. Your eyes can see the visual image of your own body getting thinner but is still unable to process that information to override what the brain has calculated for years, so it registers that you are larger than you really are. Thus, taking regular pictures and posting them everywhere—in the house, in the car, on your cell phone—is ESSENTIAL. You will be reprograming your brain to see your new image.

This body change also affects your friends and family. So be prepared. Let them know that you know what you are doing, and it is safe and healthy. Tell them, "I have decided to start treating my body in a healthy way" and *"You Can Never Go Wrong Eating Right!"*

To make a HUGE mental transformation, you really must take inventory of how you got to where you are, as well as what is your current lifestyle. It is different for each of us, but here are some things to consider from a long list of possibilities:

- Your childhood environment: Was it active, passive, sad, happy, loving, supportive?
- Your adult living environment (past and current).
- Food as a reward: Clean your plate to get dessert; candy is a treat...What were you told as a child?
- Have you gone for periods of time without access to healthy food choices or no food at all?
- The fitness and health of your close family members: Have you been living in an environment surrounded by overfat, overeating people?
- What did you learn in school about health and nutrition? Probably all the wrong things!
- Have you had significant health challenges?

- Traumatic experience(s): Have you experienced a death of a loved one, a severe accident, physical assault, a great loss, or bullying? Did food make you feel better?
- How have financial resources impacted your food choices?

By acknowledging the past triggers, and recognizing those in your current environment, you will then be able to drive the changes.

How Do You Currently Feel About Yourself?

Take out a piece of paper, at the top write "Old Me." Now start writing, just one or two words at a time, listing how you see yourself or feel about yourself.

What words are you writing? Are some of the words: *fat, ugly, disgusting? Failure, loser, stupid, out of shape?* Keep going, get them all out. Write as many as you can think of. The words you beat yourself up with every day. When you are finished, and can think of no more words, fold up the paper, take it outside and burn it (safely, of course)! They no longer exist! You do not want those thoughts anymore plaguing you and you must destroy the vibrations those words possess.

How Do You Want to See Yourself?

Now take out another piece of paper. At the top write the words "I AM." Write words on this paper of how you want to be, as if you already are: *Beautiful, fit, smart, lean, handsome, worthwhile; I am lovable and valuable just because I am me. I am wearing a size six pant. I am in a size seven dress. I am lean and riding my motorcycle again. I am able to mow the lawn without being out of breath and taking breaks. I am able to play catch with my son without knee pain. I am able to get out of bed and stand up. I am able to walk across the room without my walker. I am able to get on the floor with my grandchildren.*

Keep writing. Write as many descriptive words or phrases as you can, as if you are already there. Feel it and imagine it. When you are finished, do not fold this one up. Make copies and put them where you will see them every day. Put them on the refrigerator, your bathroom mirror, your underwear drawer, and your closet door. Somewhere you can see the words as you pass by. You can also take a picture and have it on your cell phone, so you are never without these positive words. Any place where you can frequently stop and refresh your memory with who you are now!

Read it daily, especially after you wake up in the morning and before going to bed. These are the times when your subconscious mind is receptive. These are the thoughts you are replacing in the space of your brain where the negative words used to live. **Remember: Two thoughts cannot occupy the same space in the brain.** Your new thoughts will create your own reality. Imagine yourself in this new body, moving freely. FEEL IT! Remember, feeling it will lead to thoughts and in turn you will create your own reality. Without the element of emotion, your subconscious mind cannot create the vibration for the image you want. Positive breeds positive. Just as much as negative breeds negative. So if you are going to think, think positively. After a while, you will see changes not only in yourself but all around you, within your family and with your friends. The vibrational energy from positive thoughts can help you to metabolize better and to lose fat faster. Negative becomes sluggish. FYF4Good is a Lifestyle that is all about positive. *Healthy Body, Healthy Mind!*

Coach Jennifer
Get Ready to Shift Your Paradigm!

May I just be a little candid with you? We're among friends, right? Do you have siblings? If you do, were you compared to your siblings when you were growing up? I was CONSTANTLY being compared to my siblings. And I mean CONSTANTLY.

My younger sister has an extremely high IQ, so I heard about that a LOT from Dad. I knew I was smart, however not THAT smart! But it was my other sister that I was compared to the most. When you are an identical twin, it seems to automatically give everyone else a license to study, compare, and comment on the differences (if they can find any) and similarities, that you have with your twin. Oh joy.

Until my senior year in high school, nobody knew my name except my mom and both of my sisters. To everybody else my name was "Annie-or-Jennie-whichever-you-are." Seriously! Our dad, cousins, grandparents, aunts, uncles, kids we had known since kindergarten, none of them knew who I was. So, I never had a best friend, and I never dated. Who wants to share secrets or go out on a date with someone when they don't know for sure when they are talking to her or talking to her sister? Right?

By the time we started high school, I was very self-conscious about this, so you can imagine how devastating the following experience was for me.

Ann and I went to sophomore orientation as our 10th grade year was starting. This was an opportunity to find our classes and our lockers. We also were required to go to meet our academic counselor that day. There were two of them, one for the first half of the alphabet, and one for the second half. Since we had the same last name, we had the same counselor, so we decided to go together. Might as well get the counselor used to the fact that we are twins and, yes, we DO look alike.

I can see the scene so clearly, like it happened just last week. We stood in her office. She looked from one of us, to the other, and back again. Back and forth. Studying. Finally, she said it. "I've got it. I can see the difference. One of you is a little heavier than the other." Wait. WHAT?! Time stopped. I think I stopped breathing. One of us is heavier than the other?

Later when my twin sister and I were alone, I asked the dreaded question. How much do you weigh? My heart sank. I WAS THE HEAVIER ONE. By five pounds! At fifteen that is HORRIBLE NEWS. I am crying as I type this paragraph. How could the counselor say that to a fifteen-year-old girl?

That became my self-fulfilling prophesy as those words rang through my head thousands of times over the next several years. I used them to justify eating a little more ice cream, or a few more cookies, or some extra chocolate, because, after-all, I was the heavier twin!

Each of us has a unique story regarding how we have become the person that we are. Probably all of us have experienced some hurtful negative things and, along with the happy positive things, they have helped to shape who we are, not only physically but emotionally, and mentally.

Within the mental portion is your self-image. For your metamorphosis to be complete, you must go through a transformation, a paradigm shift, of your self-image to release the negative parts and replace them with a healthy, positive image. This will take time, but it will be worth it. And those of us who have traveled this road ahead of you are here to help you along the journey. If you have close to one hundred pounds or more to lose, make sure to read chapter seven: "FYF4Good Power100 Heroes." We would be honored to walk this path with you!

THE FIRST STEPS TO A POSITIVE EMOTIONAL TRANSFORMATION

Remember that you did not get overfat overnight, so your journey to lean, optimal physical, mental, and emotional health will not happen overnight. Making the behavioral and physical transformation is a major step in all of this. Following the 8 Essential Pillars to a "T" will get you there physically the fastest and the safest. Taking the first steps toward getting lean will give you a sense of pride for taking back your life. What can you do to accelerate your mental and emotional transformation about how you see yourself?

- **Just say thank you**: When you start getting the compliments about your physical transformation, such as, "Hey it looks like you have dropped weight," and "You look nice today," or "You seem to have a healthy glow," respond by saying "Thank you." Never negate the compliment. In the past, you might have said "Oh, I am so overweight" or "No, I look horrible" or "Oh, I have so much further to go!" That's too many words! Just say "Thank you." It is okay to say, "Thank you, I really have been focusing on my health" or "Thank you for noticing." But never again negate a compliment. Why? Because first of all, when you do that you are taking the joy away from the person who just gave the kind compliment to you. And second, you reinforce a negative way of looking at yourself. Positive breeds positive.

- **Celebrate the baby steps**: Spend time each day to pat yourself on the back for at least one accomplishment. Here are some of the many things to celebrate on your journey:

   You made it through the day, the week, a month following Phase 1 to a "T."

   Your knees and ankles do not hurt as much.

   Your clothes fit looser.

   You dropped a clothing size.

   Your blood work is showing better numbers.

   You remembered to take all of your supplements.

   This week you walked a little further, a little faster, a little longer than last week.

   Celebrate something every day!

- **Develop yourself to change your mind**: Give yourself a command and follow it. That is the definition of discipline. Spend less time in front of the TV and more time developing your mind. Read positive development and attitude books, listen to CDs or pod-casts, learn new craft projects, learn a new language, go to seminars, take an FYF4Good online course, and surround yourself with people that are interested in growing in a positive way. Knowledge is power! Education and repetition will change your subconscious mind where your emotions live and thus change your old paradigms. Helping others will take the focus off you, will improve their journey, and will help you to feel thankful to have the knowledge to do so. As a bonus, you will surely make some new friends along the way. Daydream about the possibilities. And as you become a more attractive person emotionally, your vibrations will be attracting wonderful, positive changes into your life!

- **Do something for yourself:** Find your joy. Every day try to do something to make yourself feel better: If you love the garden, get out and plant something you will love to watch grow. Spend time with your animals, light a candle, diffuse essential oils, take a bubble bath, play music or paint or spend time with your kids/grandkids—whatever you like. Have fun changing your hairstyle and the colors of your clothes, or alter your make up (if you wear it). Too often we consume our lives with eating, sleeping, work, paying bills, cleaning, and laundry and miss time for ourselves. We will not get this day back. We are not promised tomorrow, ever. Honor the life that has been given to you and enjoy it. Life is to be lived. So let the living begin!

- **Have an** *"attitude of gratitude"*: It is impossible to be grateful and be depressed. In the morning, first thing, get out a piece of paper and list all the little and big things that you are grateful for. It could be that you are grateful for an unusually delicious, frothy FYF4Good Latte, or your good health, your home, your food, your family, your dog, finding the FYF4Good Lifestyle, etc.! You understand. See how many of the tiniest things you can list that you are grateful for. It will surely put you in to what we call an *"attitude of gratitude"* and thankfulness, which is a very peaceful place to be and should make you smile. This in turn will create the vibration that will be a magnet for positive things to happen.

- **Enjoy the little things:** Have you ever heard of the saying "Stop and smell the roses"? Every day, even if it is just ten seconds here or a minute there, start to take this time. It is easy. Before you start to drink your coffee, take a minute to smell it. When you eat your food, take time to chew a few of the mouthfuls more slowly, tasting and enjoying the texture of the food in your mouth. When you walk out of the house in the morning, stop for one minute and listen to the birds singing. Before going to bed, check on your sleeping child and listen to his or her breath. Walk outside and enjoy the sunset or look up at the stars. Amazing! Find time throughout the day to consciously do this. Every day. They say a man gets his best ideas mowing the lawn. Why? He gave his brain a break and focused on a physical activity. It is all about balance.

- **Care about how you look:** Start walking the walk. Get out of the sweat pants! As you lose the fat you need to immediately start dressing as a "fit, healthy person." Get rid of the baggy clothes, the extra sizes in the closet. Donate or throw out baggy T-shirts, sweat pants, worn-out clothes. Shop at second-hand stores as you are rapidly transitioning through sizes. You can find brand new clothes (with department store tags still on them), and like-new clothes at these stores for very reasonable prices. Wearing new clothes will change the way you see yourself, as well as the way others see you.

  Take pride in how you look, every day! If you are in your forties or older and still have the same haircut you had in high school, guess what? This is the old you. It is time for a change. Cut or style your hair differently. Color the gray, wear makeup, shave, manicure, pedicure … fix it up! Create a fresh new you!

- **Tear down the camouflage; get out of your comfort zone:** As we have become overfat, we find ways to hide our true selves behind that. It may mean we have become the jokester, the life of the party, making jokes about ourselves. Our camouflage may be that we do not leave the house; we limit our time around others. Maybe we wear black all the time to look smaller. Or we wear baggy clothes. To make drastic changes in our lives, we need to make drastic changes. If you are doing things the same old way, ask yourself why you are doing them (and how is that working for you?) If the answer is not a healthy, positive reason, then STOP! Do something different. Discipline yourself on a new path. Only when you choose to take the other path, will you get to a new place. Every day on FYF4Good is a day you can feel good about yourself. Again, give yourself a command and follow it. That is the true meaning of discipline.

- **Be selfish with your time**: If you have family members, friends, coworkers, or neighbors that make you feel bad, start limiting your time with them. This negative energy is not healthy. We each are given only so many minutes in our lifetime. You are now on a journey, the FYF4Good journey, to become lean and healthy for life, so that you can enjoy your life. Do not let anything or anyone get in your way. You will never get the time back that is wasted on negative people. Get out and meet new people: volunteer for a nonprofit, join a church or synagogue, attend a Sunday school group, take a class, find a new walking group, join a meet-up, or go to a self-help or personal development class or to a seminar. Spend your time meeting new people that you can enjoy being around, and stay close to those who are investing in your success. These are the kind of people you will find in the Private Flush Your Fat 4Good "Buddies" Facebook Group. Get to know your Buddies there!

- **Love yourself:** If you are like most of us when we started this journey, you may hate yourself. You do not like who you have become, the way you look, the way you feel. You probably have felt this way for a very long time. Feeling different is a conscious choice. You will continue to feel this way until you make a commitment in your mind, a conscious effort to change it. By doing so, you will instigate the good emotions in your subconscious. Assume now you are who you want to become. Before you know it, it will be effortless. To feel freedom from the darkness of those negative thoughts will lead to your quest for joy and expansion will be your existential results. Bookmark this chapter. Reread it frequently. Monthly, weekly, daily: Do whatever it takes to evolve your mind to a healthy place.

Through regularly thinking positive thoughts about how you feel, what you look like and who you are, guess what will happen? One day you will wake up and no longer have to consciously make this effort because you will be living it! So act as if you are there already.

As Dr. Vicky always says, *"Stay the course. Trust the process!"*

CHAPTER NINE

FYF4GOOD STAPLES

Jackie's Chicken Salad, FYF4Good Latte, Goat Yogurt with Nuts, organic coffee, healthy milks and fruits, and other delicious stuff

FYF4Good is *Health by Design, Not by Default!* What does that mean? It means your body was designed by God, and it should be fed the way it was designed to be fed. But our default has become fast foods, processed foods, and meal replacement shakes and bars. The shortcuts of life are killing us.

On Phase 1 it is recommended that you eat at least five servings of Jackie's Chicken Salad every week. Why Jackie's Chicken Salad and not chicken salad from the grocery store? Why do we drink organic coffee, one to three cups every day? Why goat yogurt with nuts? Why? Because we are striving for optimal health. This Lifestyle was designed with details to help us all get as close to it as possible, as quickly as possible.

JACKIE'S CHICKEN SALAD

*Jackie's Chicken Salad should be a **staple**. Whenever you are hungry, you have got to eat something. Tupperware should be your best friend. Rip up some kale in the bottom of a Tupperware container and throw in a little handful of arugula. Dump a soup ladle of Jackie's Chicken Salad on top of it. Put the lid on, grab a spoon, and run out the door. That is how it should be. It should always be available.*—Jackie Padgette-Baird

Jackie's Chicken Salad Recipe
(four to five servings)

Ingredients

One whole organic free-range chicken or two to three skinned, boneless, organic free-range chicken breasts

Two to three dill pickles, diced into small pieces

Two to three medium organic cucumbers (Persian cucumbers are GREAT), chopped into small pieces

One tomato, cut into small pieces *(optional)*

One cup broccoli florets, finely chopped

Two to three rounded tablespoons organic, unsweetened, non-GMO, EDTA-free mayonnaise

One shallot, finely chopped

Juice from two to three large lemons

Pink Himalayan Salt

Extra virgin cold-pressed pure olive oil (no blended olive oil)

Montreal Steak Seasoning (find at Costco)

No-Salt Seasoning (find at Costco)

Preparation

Wash the chicken breasts thoroughly. Either leave them whole or cut length wise as tenders.

Heat olive oil in the bottom of a grill pan *(a grill pan is best and is easy to find if you do not have one)* and lightly sprinkle Montreal Steak Seasoning and Organic No-Salt Seasoning on top of the oil. Get the oil really hot and then sear the chicken breasts (or tenders). Grill on both sides until they are golden brown. It is a delicious taste when prepared this way! Let the chicken cool and chop it into little bite size pieces in a large bowl. Mix in the chopped cucumbers.

When eating broccoli, a cruciferous vegetable, we recommend lightly steaming to facilitate digestion. However for this salad, finely chop the raw florets (not the stems) and add to the bowl.

Add two to three rounded tablespoons of mayonnaise to the bowl.

Squeeze the juice from two to three (*sometimes four depending on their size*) lemons into the bowl. You may always add more lemon if desired.

Add the finely chopped shallot and the diced dill pickles to the bowl.

Add the chopped tomatoes (*optional*).

Season with Pink Himalayan Salt to taste.

Mix well.

Refrigerate and have available with a bag of kale and arugula right next to it.

To Serve

When hungry, grab a handful of kale and a handful of arugula; rinse and throw them in a bowl or on a dinner plate. Take a large heaping soup ladle of Jackie's Chicken Salad and place on top. Convenience and easy access is VERY important! YUM!

Deep Dive into "why" we choose Jackie's Chicken Salad *There is a method to her madness!*

Jackie's Chicken Salad is loaded with protein! Why is protein so important? It is one of the main building blocks for our bones, blood, tissue, muscles, cartilage, skin and hair, and the repair of our organs. Protein is very important for helping to build our lean muscle mass. Strong muscles help us burn fat more efficiently and quickly. Protein is also very important for blood sugar stabilization and regulation.

Other proteins (turkey, egg, salmon, tuna, sardines, other fish, grass-fed beef, lamb, tofu or Spice of Life Meatless Meats if vegan) can be substituted in the Jackie's Chicken Salad recipe for variety from time to time, but the best choice for Jackie's Chicken Salad is ... well ... CHICKEN. Take a look at what chicken has to offer!

Chicken has l-lysine and l-arginine. These are two amino acids that are important for healing and are building blocks for our bodies. Chicken also has one of the highest contents of leucine, as well as isoleucine, and valine which are branched-chain amino acids (BCAA's). The BCAA's are extremely effective to help you build lean muscle, while burning the fat.

Jackie's Egg Salad is easier to make. Hard boil the eggs, let them cool, and make your salad with the recipe earlier in this section, chopping up the eggs rather than the grilled chicken. There is a protein called albumin contained in the white of the eggs. It is necessary to maintain good health. (Notice on a comprehensive blood test, you will see levels of albumin tested in the blood.) The whole egg is the perfect source of protein. A little mustard in this salad is delicious!

Dark Meat versus White Meat

White meat (breast, wings) has more lysine. There is less fat in the white meat. The dark meat (legs) contains more iron, which is why it is darker. Chicken contains high phosphorus, selenium, niacin, and vitamins B6 and B12 with the skin.

You can choose to use either white or dark (or both) meat in your Jackie's Chicken Salad. It is all in the taste. Just about every part of the chicken has health benefits to it. Even the liver and gizzards are okay if the chicken was not eating tainted feed, is pesticide-free, and has roamed the range. Buy organically raised, free-range chickens. Free-range means these chickens are eating the bugs off the ground. Chickens are supposed to eat bugs, not grains. When they do, they produce eggs, and the next generation of chickens, that contain higher omega-3 fatty acid content. This is good!

Some people believe that the chicken's skin should be avoided, but this is not true. In nature, all protein is accompanied by fat. The skin is the fat. It has CLA (Conjugated Linolenic Acid) in it. When eating the skin, you should also be eating the meat. Do not go wild eating much more skin than is contained on your piece of meat, as it will challenge your gallbladder. The recipe for Jackie's Chicken Salad leaves the skin out; however you can include the skin if desired.

What about the cucumber?

There are a lot of wonderful things in cucumbers including phytosterols (plant hormones) and high levels of vitamin C. Cucumbers are a fruit vegetable, like a tomato, because they have seeds. It is a low-glycemic, watery, crispy vegetable with anticancer properties and excellent phytonutrients. Cucumbers are crunchy, fresh, and they do not interfere with the taste of the salad. Organic is preferred when possible, as commercial cucumbers are highly sprayed with pesticides.

> *I could have used zucchini instead of cucumber in Jackie's Chicken Salad, but it did not work. It did not have the fresh fluid concept to it.*
> —Jackie Padgette-Baird

Broccoli, the Power Veggie

Broccoli, a cruciferous vegetable, should ordinarily be slightly steamed or grilled before eating because it is easier to digest when you break up the fibrous content. Since we are only eating the florets, we do not need to steam it. Organic broccoli is considered one of the most balanced vegetables. Cruciferous vegetables are proactive in the body to fight cancers and help to boost the immune system. Wonderful benefits for EVERYONE!

Lemon and Mayo

Lemons are acidic but have an alkaline effect in the body; the juice cuts (helps to emulsify) the fats, stimulates salivation, cleanses the liver and gallbladder, marinates, and is a natural preservative. Lemon juice helps to break down the broccoli, the cellulose in the greens and other vegetables, as well as the meat. Our bodies are unable to break down cellulose. Lemon is the very best alternative to using vinegar. Most Buddies never ever go back to vinegar, even while eating on Phase 2, once they have been using lemon juice. The mayonnaise is additional fat that gives the salad a nice creamy texture and curtails the sourness of the lemon juice. A nutritional benefit of mayonnaise is that the oils are necessary for the lutein and the zeaxanthin to be absorbed from your greens. These nutrients are extremely beneficial for the health of the macula in the eye, and may prevent macular degeneration, the leading cause of blindness in the elderly.

Be sure to read the label and pick a mayonnaise that has no sugar or EDTA. If you visit a blood lab, almost every vial of blood contains a preservative called EDTA (short for ethylene diamine tetra-acetic acid). It is a chemical that is not normally found in human blood but enters the body through the foods we eat. It is not good for the body because it prevents blood from clotting. When mixed in a sealed vial, EDTA can keep a blood sample liquid for years. You will be amazed when reading the labels of foods you have bought over the years. Many have EDTA in them. FYF4Good facilitates the body to remove chemicals and toxins from our bodies. Therefore, to continue to ingest chemicals and toxins makes no sense.

Onions (Shallots) and Pickles for More than Flavor

Onions have a lot of great health benefits. There is a phytochemical called allicin and there is plenty in shallot onions. This is a sulfur compound, which possesses antioxidant activity and has shown a variety of actions potentially very useful for human health. Allicin exhibits hypolipidemic, antiplatelet, and pro-circulatory effects. Allicin also contains antibacterial and cancer-preventive properties. Onions contain sulfur that is excellent nutrition for the joints. And since onions are pro-circulatory, they are also very good for your heart. And for allergy sufferers, a study has shown supplements containing allicin reduce allergic symptoms such as coughing and sneezing. Why not eat a little every day of your life?

> *I chose shallots because they are thinner, smaller, and daintier. They do not overwhelm the taste of your salad. If you are not crazy about onions, use shallots. When you chop them up, there will not be an overwhelming flavor in the salad. You could also use a Bermuda or another onion. Onions have a lot of fluid. This helps with the texture and fluidity for digestion of the salad.* —Jackie Padgette-Baird

Dill pickles are made from cucumbers. Do not drink the dill pickle juice. It contains vinegar which is great for preserving the pickles but is not something we consume in Phase 1. Vinegar promotes the growth of yeast, and most people who need to lose fat need to get rid of the yeast that disrupts the balance of good and bad bacteria in the body that can slow down metabolism and contribute to weight gain. The process of **lacto-fermentation** happens when the starches and sugars within the cucumber are converted to lactic acid by the friendly bacteria lactobacilli. So the term **"lacto"** in lacto-fermentation actually refers to this production of lactic acid, not **lacto** as in the lactose in milk. This is what promotes salivation and serves a purpose to aid digestion. Do not ever eat sweet pickles. They contain sugar which will stop digestion!

> *Most people use sweet relish or sweet pickles in salads such as tuna salad, egg salad, and chicken salad. NO! We are not doing anything sweet, and the reason I wanted the dill pickle is it has a sour, tart taste. It has phytosterols in it, which is interesting. Even though we are not eating a lot of these in the salad, it is really nice to add this to counteract the deficiency of our Lifestyle. The dill pickle also stimulates salivation. When you chew on the salad and you have a little piece of dill pickle in there, you start to salivate again. Your juices in your mouth come out. This creates better mastication. Same with the lemon!* —Jackie Padgette-Baird

Kale and Arugula

We serve the chicken salad on a bed of kale and arugula. They were picked for their nutritional value. Both are cruciferous vegetables, which we cannot get enough of. Kale has important phytochemicals and carotenoids and lutein for eye health. These greens also contain good amounts of magnesium and potassium. If you find you are having cramping, re-evaluate whether you are eating enough greens. If not, eat more!

Arugula is an aphrodisiac. Believe it or not, after eating Jackie's Chicken Salad, emotionally the salad puts you into a euphoric moment of feeling really good and completely satisfied. The arugula adds a peppery, spicy taste, another distinct flavor that makes for the deliciousness of the salad. The older and larger the leaves, the more peppery taste they have. All of these flavors combine perfectly together.

There are different kinds of kale. Some are big and tough. Some are small, like the arugula. So, try different kinds if you do not like the first one you try, and have fun experimenting with the different flavors and textures that kale has to offer. Be sure to remove the heavy steams, as these are difficult to digest raw and can be woody. For those concerned about their blood clotting medication, please talk with your health care practitioner. Make sure you are being monitored regularly and let him or her know that the kale and the broccoli are in small amounts.

Summary of Jackie's Chicken Salad

Every flavor in Jackie's Chicken Salad tantalizes your taste buds. You do not get bored with it because all of those different flavors hit different parts of your tongue in different ways. And it creates a desire to eat more.

People have found that when they eat Jackie's Chicken Salad on a daily basis, they lose more fat than when they do not eat it daily. There really is something magical about this recipe.

You should always have Jackie's Chicken Salad available, especially on Phase 1. Have up to three or four days of salad ready in the refrigerator at all times. Instead of Jackie's Three-Egg Omelet or goat yogurt with nuts in the morning, you can have a bowl of Jackie's Chicken Salad. It picks you up, gives you a lot of energy, and it really sustains your energy for a long time.

It is amazing how there are absolutely no cravings for anything else after you have had your fill of Jackie's Chicken Salad.

So many times I will have my fruit, wait twenty minutes, and then make my FYF4Good Latte. Then about thirty to forty minutes after that I find myself hungry. It is time to listen to my brain. And especially the different weathers will determine how you feel and what you want and need to eat. Many days, I just say, 'You know what, I am hungry. I am going to have that chicken salad now instead of eggs, because it is what I was hearing my body tell me. Listen to your health-conscious brain. It does wonders.
—Jackie Padgette-Baird

JACKIE'S THREE-EGG OMELET

If you want a three-egg omelet every morning, eat it! But wait a minute, isn't eating too many eggs bad for you? That is an old paradigm. We were raised with that belief, but there is now new research. The cholesterol in the yolk is essential for the emulsification of the white. The yolk of the egg is loaded with lecithin, which is important for our brain, lungs, heart, and nerves. There is also a lot of lutein in the yolk which greatly benefits eye health. Eating the whole egg is essential. It is the perfect protein. Why not eat eggs several times a week? With all those benefits, it is awesome to feed your body eggs!

Emma Morano, age 116, from Verbania, Italy, was the oldest living person. Ms. Morano died May 11, 2016. In an interview in 2015, she told the *New York Times* that she attributes the secret to her longevity to eating three raw eggs every single day since her teens. She was told to eat raw eggs by her doctor after being diagnosed with anemia. The math would calculate Ms. Morano would have consumed about one hundred and ten thousand (110,000) eggs in her lifetime, including the cholesterol.

Cooking Omelets

Heat up the oil, whisk three eggs, and cook (like a flat pancake) on one side. Flip the eggs over and pile on chopped up vegetables (yellow and orange peppers, mushrooms, kale, broccoli tops, asparagus, or whatever you like) down the middle. Add a little goat cheese, fold the egg over (like a taco), grate pecorino sheep cheese on top, cover and let steam. This will soften the vegetables and melt the cheese. YUM!!

Cooking Jackie's Egg and Veggie Muffins

Beat up twelve eggs. Cut up vegetables, such as red bell peppers, asparagus, chopped broccoli tops, onions, mushrooms, zucchini, kale, and arugula. Make the vegetables pieces small.

Spray coconut or olive oil into the muffin holes of a twelve-hole muffin tin. Fill each of the holes with a variety of the chopped up vegetables. Take a soup ladle and pour the beaten eggs into each hole. Place a dollop of goat cheese in the middle, put a teaspoon of fresh salsa, and add grated pecorino sheep cheese on top of the salsa. Jackie loves Trader Joe's Hatch Valley Salsa. Bake at 350 degrees for approximately eighteen to twenty minutes. Pull out of the oven and let cool. They will be puffy until cool and then will slightly shrink. Keep them in a Tupperware container in the refrigerator. When you are ready to eat, just slightly steam them. They heat up very quickly, or they are also great cold.

Choosing a Good Cooking Oil

There are issues with some cooking oils. They might say they are olive oil, but they are not always just olive oil. You have to read the label really carefully. Stay away from olive oil that says "Extra virgin BLENDED olive oil." "Blended" means it is cut with vegetable oil, canola oil, or grapeseed oil, etc. Blended oils will be cheaper because they have other cheap oils mixed with the olive oil. One oil we recommend is the Costco Kirkland Organic Extra Virgin Olive Oil that has been rated as "authentic," is high quality, and tastes great.

There are a few oils to choose that are considered authentic, meaning that it is what it says it is. Organic is always the best choice. Cold-pressed and first-pressed oils are preferred. Make sure the brand of oil comes from a reputable company. Olive oil, avocado oil, and organic coconut oil are good, but make sure they are authentic. Read the label. Read the label. Read the label. Do your homework!

Or you can use butter! Do you remember when "they" told us butter was bad for your body? Buy margarine, we were told! Ugh! Margarine will wreak havoc with your health. Butter is better, but buy only organic grass-fed butter if possible!

When I am fixing my three-egg omelet, I will take a teaspoon of coconut oil and put that in the pan and then lick the spoon because I love coconut oil! It has a lot of GREAT health benefits in it. It also adds a unique flavor to my three-egg omelet. You are using it as an added benefit, but you do not want your foods to be soaking in it.— Jackie Padgette-Baird

COFFEE

Coffee is one of the highest pesticide-sprayed crops in the world, so ALWAYS choose organic coffee. The pesticides on the coffee have been the culprit that gives coffee a bad rap. Many times, it is the pesticides on the coffee that will hype you up or make you feel sick. The pesticides can actually make you feel nauseous. Besides the toxins, it is what people have put in their coffees on a daily basis that are so damaging. When you see whipped creams, half and half, artificial creamers (contains partially hydrogenated oils), sweeteners, syrups, and more, coupled with the desire to add sugar to coffee every day, this becomes a recipe for poor nutrition and is very fattening.

But coffee has MANY health benefits, when you choose organic, non-GMO, coffee. Both medium and dark roast coffees are great. If you are not accustomed to coffee, or if you are easily affected by caffeine, then pick dark roast as there are lower levels of caffeine in the dark and espresso roast coffees. Dark is roasted longer and some of the caffeine is roasted out.

You can have one to three cups a day. The health benefits are now known to be huge! Coffee is mandatory on FYF4Good. Most people who hear this cannot believe it. Unless you have a religious reason to abstain, we recommend that you drink coffee. If you have never had coffee or you do not regularly drink it, start with one-quarter of a cup in your FYF4Good Latte. There has been so much incorrect information about the adverse effects of coffee, but if you really look at the studies of the effects of coffee itself, you will find it is very beneficial to the body.

In 2015 there were two extensive studies of drinking coffee. One concluded that coffee helps prevent breast cancer and the second showed it helps prevent melanoma. Since then, more studies have come out showing prevention of other cancers as well. Other studies have been done that indicate how coffee will help a person to live longer. Here are some of the most recent facts from these studies:

- Coffee is a mood elevator.
- Coffee brings up your alertness and your IQ! It actually makes you smarter! Who cannot benefit from that?!
- Coffee helps to establish better metabolism, and it instigates your bowels to move.
- Coffee acts like a diuretic. Also as a dilator to improve breathing for people with asthma.
- Coffee is a good source of B vitamins (B1, B2, B3 and B5).
- Coffee has a concentrated source of phytochemical antioxidants. In the Western diet, it is the highest source of antioxidants.
- Coffee can make you really happy in the morning or anytime during the day. It kicks in your adrenals.
- Coffee time is a very relaxing and pleasant ritual.
- Studies are showing coffee may increase lifespan!
- BUT ... COFFEE MUST BE ORGANIC!

Is caffeine addictive?

If you overdo the number of cups of coffee, yes, it can be addictive. On FYF4Good we recommend one to three cups of coffee a day. This amount has not been shown to be an issue. Coffee is recommended by the Mayo Clinic because it provides health benefits. These benefits include a reduction in the occurrence of many health conditions as well as being one of the best-known sources of antioxidants. Up to four hundred milligrams (mg) of caffeine a day appears to be safe for most healthy adults. That is roughly the amount of caffeine in four cups of brewed coffee. Over four cups may put stress on your adrenal glands and your heart. It can also disrupt your sleep and your digestion. So, stick to one to three cups. The only addictive thing about one to three cups of coffee is all the benefits received from drinking it!

Warning: Be careful of Cuban coffee, which is usually served in thimble-like shots. It is extremely strong and is not organic. Over consumption of these "shots" of Cuban coffee can give you excessive amounts of caffeine that may have noticeable side effects in the body. It is a better idea not to consume Cuban coffee, and if you do, one shot is the limit!

WHY NO COW DAIRY?

When most of us think of yogurt, we think of COW yogurt. Cow milk (including A1 and A2), and foods made from cow milk, including cow cheese, are not the best foods for humans. It is very important for you to understand this. Our world has taught us that "Milk does a body good!" However, cow dairy has very long amino chains making up the protein in the milk. Humans cannot break down and digest these amino chains. Only calves can break apart these proteins into peptides and amino acids for digestion. Additionally, cow milk is usually pasteurized and heated to very high temperature, thereby killing enzymes, active probiotics, and anything live or beneficial in the milk. Essentially it is a dead food.

Think about it! Cow milk is designed to take a baby calf and help it grow to a one-ton animal with three stomachs. There are many growth hormones naturally present in cow milk, and humans do not digest them properly. Even if the cow has not been given hormones, the cow has its own hormones. Cow milk is not even close to human mother's milk; thus it creates a lot of health problems for babies and children.

Cow milk is very mucus-forming because of the fact that the large amino acid chains are not effectively broken down by humans for digestion. If you drink enough cow milk, the calcium in the milk has a tendency to bond with iron. This can cause you to become iron deficient and create an iron deficiency anemia. Be especially cautious with children and cow milk. Even a calf is weaned off the cow milk after about a year; they do not consume it their entire life. If you really think about it, all of this makes sense and will cause you to experience a huge Paradigm Shift in your milk choices, especially when it comes to your children!

Some people say, "I don't have any cow milk except maybe some cheese." Think again! It takes a gallon of milk to make a brick of cheese. Cow milk and cheese very commonly cause allergy issues in many people for all the reasons mentioned previously. Approximately 65 percent of the human population has a reduced ability to digest lactose after infancy. In people of East Asian descent, the reduced tolerance for lactose in adulthood affects 90 percent in some of these communities. With FYF4Good YOU WILL GET OFF COW MILK DAIRY PRODUCTS 4GOOD!

FYF4GOOD RECOMMENDED MILKS
Organic Soy Milk

Organic, unsweetened, plain, non–GMO soy milk is recommended for our FYF4Good Latte. It has seven to twelve grams of protein per cup, making it the preferred milk of choice for your FYF4Good Latte. The soy milk will give your body outstanding protein, has cancer fighting phytochemicals, is a good source of calcium, iron, riboflavin, vitamin B-12, and much more. More importantly, soy milk has been shown to be successful with rapid fat loss.

There are those who still object to soy milk, claiming that it causes thyroid issues and other hormonal issues. This is old information from a study that was done with GMO soy. There are dozens of studies on soy that disprove this information. Organic, unsweetened, plain, non–GMO soy milk is very beneficial to the body.

Goat milk is also a good choice and has about eleven grams of protein. Goat milk is the closest milk to human breast milk. You can use hemp or flax milk although the protein content is not as high. Make sure it is pure hemp or flax, not a blended liquid with sugars and other additives such as starch or a pea protein. Do not use almond milk or coconut milk as these have very little protein content, if any at all! We are looking for milks with the most protein available for our FYF4Good Latte.

Again, soy milk, MUST be organic, unsweetened, plain, non-GMO. The only sugar you should see is the small amount in the soy bean itself. Read the ingredients carefully. Sometimes "no sugar added" does not exclude other sweeteners. Make sure it is UNSWEETENED. Most vanilla milks have added sugar. If you can find one that you are sure does not have added sugar, it should be fine. No chocolate. Remember, if you see any sugar at all on the label, other than what is in the soy beans, or you are not sure of the sugar content, do not buy it. Take a picture of the nutrition label and post it in the Facebook Group. We will help you read the label.

Goat or Sheep Yogurt

With FYF4Good, the recommended yogurt is goat, but sheep yogurt is also good. Yogurt has live probiotics and it benefits our entire digestive tract. Probiotics support a strong immune system (because 70 to 80 percent of your immune system is in your gut) and will improve health. It is all about the gut! Because digestion and absorption are improved, goat or sheep yogurt supports fat loss.

Some people complain that they do not like the flavor of goat or sheep yogurt, but keep in mind that it takes ten days to reprogram the taste buds. Many Buddies have found this to be true and overtime they suddenly miss it if they do not have it! It is so worth it to work on acquiring the taste to make goat or sheep yogurt part of the foods in your life. Stick with it, and you will develop many new healthy habits with this Lifestyle. The sheep yogurt has a sharper taste and more protein in it. Jackie loves mixing them both together for a unique flavor. Check out the section "How to Find a New Taste You Love in Ten Days" in chapter eleven to learn how to love goat yogurt.

Additionally, goat and sheep dairy have fewer allergenic proteins and cause less inflammation. The goat and sheep cheeses are delicious adding flavor in omelets with chopped up vegetables or to a salad.

*When I chose goat yogurt, I wanted something that was going to be unique. I wanted a different taste. I wanted something that was going to be creamy, something that was going to have health benefits. But also something that was going to be a little different and that would be special—And then when I put the nuts in the goat yogurt I said— Aha! Everybody who has been on this Lifestyle for some time knows that there's a moment when they say, 'I've got to have that chicken salad' and there are other moments when they say, 'I've got to have my goat yogurt with nuts!' —*Jackie Padgette-Baird

GOAT YOGURT WITH NUTS
Why Do We Eat Goat or Sheep Yogurt With Nuts?

Eating goat yogurt plain, by putting it in your mouth and swallowing it, is like drinking it. There is no chewing. When you put a handful of walnuts, pecans, or seeds into the yogurt, it makes you have to "chew" your yogurt. Remember, *The Harder to Chew, the More You Lose!* We also want to encourage a slower time in eating and absorption of foods for better digestion. Additionally, the nuts are added protein, they contain live enzymes (enzymes aid digestion), and the oils in the nuts are extremely beneficial. Not to mention that it helps your blood sugar to remain stable. You will find that you enjoy eating the yogurt with nuts and are surprisingly satisfied. It becomes a meal to sustain you.

We mandate eating goat yogurt with nuts and seeds pretty much every single day. There are many benefits gained from eating goat or sheep yogurt. The probiotic and nutritional benefits are tremendous because they help to maximize a healthy gut, lower the risk of diabetes, support weight and fat loss, and may even help to reduce high blood pressure.

We have found that goat yogurt with nuts are extremely convenient to take on the go in a plastic container. If you feel that you are not very hungry and would like something lighter than a protein and vegetable meal or Jackie's Chicken Salad, goat yogurt with nuts is the perfect choice. Alternatively, if you feel like you could eat more after your protein and vegetable meal, you can have your goat yogurt with nuts approximately one hour or more after eating your protein meal to enjoy it as a "dessert."

Basically, we want to keep the metabolism fired up and burning fat. Goat yogurt with nuts is so good that you will find yourself craving it. By keeping the metabolism and your blood sugar stable, there will not be any spikes or dips and you will have sustained energy from the stored fat you continue to burn. It is like putting the kindling on the campfire when the fire starts to burn out.

Some people will put the goat yogurt with nuts into the freezer for a short period of time before eating. It reminds them of ice cream. A lot of people add cinnamon to the yogurt and nut mix, but it is good to also learn to eat the yogurt plain with just the nuts/seeds. *Let Your Brain Enjoy Plain!*

When you do not have nuts on hand or you want to mix it up a little, slice up some cucumber, Bermuda red onions and a sprinkle of dill weed in your yogurt. It is delicious!

Remember to wait four hours after you finish eating any protein before you have fruit.

NUTS AND SEEDS
WHICH ONES ARE GOOD FOR US?

In the United States, most almonds are grown in California and after the E. coli scare, all raw almonds organic or conventional must be pasteurized by law. Pasteurization involves heating and/or gassing the raw almonds to kill any E.coli that might be contaminating the nuts. We do not want to eat pasteurized raw almonds or any other pasteurized nuts, because they cannot be brought to life by soaking. Eating pasteurized nuts also involves the digestion of chemicals that we do not want to ingest into our bodies. Therefore, we recommend that you purchase organic raw almonds grown in Europe or other places around the world that do not pasteurize the nuts. You can find these vendors online and conveniently have them shipped to your doorstep.

Do not be fooled by packages of raw, organic cashews. They have also been pasteurized. So, they are dead, and you do not want that. You want raw, organic nuts that are from a reputable company. Check the labels on packages; regulations require disclosure if they are pasteurized.

Walnuts are excellent nuts to choose because of the omega-3 fatty acids contained in them. You also receive wonderful protein and beneficial phytonutrients from walnuts. Pecans are another awesome choice. They have great phytonutrient value. Another absolutely delicious raw nut to have in your goat yogurt is organic raw macadamia nuts. Scrumptious!

Pretty much any raw soaked nuts or seeds that you would like to have in your goat or sheep yogurt is a go! Peanuts are not a nut, so do not eat them. They are a legume, a bean, and therefore a starch. One caution: Pine nuts are great and so good for your immune system, but frequently eating too many of them could possibly result in a metallic taste in the mouth. It will go away, but this is very annoying. Been there, done that! A handful of nuts in each serving of goat or sheep yogurt are about the right amount.

All seeds are terrific, and soaked pumpkin seeds are fantastic when you prepare them with this recipe that Jackie developed. Soak and dry the pumpkin seeds *(keep reading to learn how)*. Then spray them with coconut oil and sprinkle them with Pink Himalayan Salt *(optional)* and sprinkle on some cayenne pepper. Put them back in the oven for about another hour at 170 degrees Fahrenheit. This will dry the oil, causing the cayenne pepper and the salt to stick to the seeds. YUM! This is a treat that you can munch on while watching a movie or add to your yogurt. By the way, you can also eat your goat yogurt with a combination of nuts and seeds. How healthy is that to have every day!

There is one seed we do not have to soak: hemp seed. This seed has GREAT amounts of omega-3, and omega-6 fatty acids. Hemp seeds are chewy, very delicious, with a nutty taste and very high in protein.

Why soak the nuts?

Those that say they cannot eat nuts most likely have never soaked them. Nuts contain phytates, which by definition is phytic acid bound to a mineral. The phytic acid binds to the mineral in the nut, seed, grain, or legume, and this phytate is the energy source for sprouting the nut or seed to get it to come to life. In simple terms, a nut is a seed: it has a shell on it, it is hard, and it is dormant. In nature, when the nut falls to the ground and comes into contact with water, the soil and the minerals in the soil, as well as the heat of the sun will cause it to sprout.

The problem is that phytic acid can also bind with minerals in the human gut before they are absorbed, and they can negatively influence the digestive enzymes. The mineral zinc, for example, is a mineral that is necessary to make digestive enzymes in the body. Zinc, as well as other minerals, are leached out of the body when the phytates are not removed. Phytates can reduce the digestion of proteins, carbohydrates, starches, and fats. Soaking the nuts overnight with Pink Himalayan Salt, draining and rinsing thoroughly, and also using low heat (150-170 degree oven) to dry the nuts (not to roast them) must be done to remove phytates.

Raw, unsoaked nuts are hard to digest. If you are used to eating the soaked nuts, and then you eat them unsoaked, you will not be able to eat as many. You will feel it in your stomach and gut. Most phytates are degraded in the stomach and small intestine. This will create discomfort when your digestive enzymes are compromised, and minerals will leave the body by attaching themselves to the phytic acid. For these reasons, raw nuts, seeds, grains, and legumes all need to be soaked before consuming them. Many people do not like to eat nuts because it hurts their gut. They are missing out on incredible nutrition.

For those who are concerned about the salt, think again.... There is no salt in soaked nuts. When you soak nuts and rinse and dry them, they are not salty. The salt provides the media for a chemical reaction to take the phytates out and ignite the nut to life. The residue is rinsed away with the phytates. There are minerals in the soil that do the same thing in nature. When it rains, the water reacts with the minerals in the soil.

Why Pink Himalayan Salt?

FYF4Good recommends Pink Himalayan Salt. We do not recommend iodized, regular, table salt. Table salt is processed. It has no minerals in it. It is sodium and chloride. It is not salt in its complete form that includes all the wonderful minerals and trace minerals that natural sea salt contains.

Pink Himalayan Salt is NOT processed. It is dried in the sun in its natural form. Sea Salt contains chlorine, sodium, sulfur, magnesium, potassium, carbon as carbonic acid, bromine, baron, and strontium. There are more than forty "minor elements" including every known or unknown trace element of nutritional significance. It is postulated that there are eighty-four natural minerals in Pink Himalayan Salt. This large concentration of minerals includes calcium, potassium, magnesium, and sulfur, which are deficient in the American diet. If you cannot find the Pink Himalayan Salt, look for Celtic Sea Salt or an unprocessed naturally dried sea salt. You will get the same benefit, but by all means, do not use iodized processed table salt. Eat salt to your taste. Your brain will be in charge.

What about Roasted Nuts?

Every protein is accompanied by a fat. When you roast nuts you remove the fat and denature the whole nut. The good fat is roasted out, and bad fats and processed salt are added. It is practically a carbohydrate at this point because it really does not react like a protein in the body. It is dead. You have roasted it and now it is dried out and it goes to sugar in the digestive tract. Do not eat roasted nuts! It is just common sense!

Busting a Myth about Peanuts

A lot of people need to understand that peanuts are not a nut. They are a legume. They are a bean or what is called a goober. Peanuts are a STARCH! We do not eat starches on FYF4Good Phase 1. Peanuts and legumes are great with grains; therefore enjoy them in Phase 2. And, again, if they are roasted, the beneficial oils have been removed, and processed salt has been added. Roasted peanuts are a bad recipe for colon problems. Raw, organic peanuts or raw peanut butter are okay when on Phase 2. They require a two-hour digestion time because they are a starch. However, be very picky with your peanuts and peanut butter as they can contain a carcinogen called aflatoxin, a natural toxin produced by certain strains of the mold aspergillus flavus and A. parasiticus that grow on peanuts stored in warm, humid silos.

LOW-GLYCEMIC ORGANIC FRUITS AND VEGETABLES

Whenever you eat fruit, it is important to choose fruit that is in season. Our bodies perform differently depending on the seasons and will "run" better with the fruits and vegetables in season. The seasonal fruits will not only taste better, but they will have the most nutrients. If you are in Phase 2 and enjoying sweet melons, remember that melons should always be eaten alone or with other melons. They do not digest well with other fruits.

Additionally, citrus fruits such as oranges, grapefruits and tangerines are also Phase 2 fruits and do not digest well in combination with other fruit.

Always choose organic fruits and vegetables when possible and wash them thoroughly before consuming. We are trying to remove all pesticides and toxins from our bodies, so it is important to not put any more in.

Why do we eat fruit as our breakfast first thing in the morning?

If you treat your body correctly it will work like clockwork. The assimilation cycle is 8:00 p.m. to 4:00 a.m. All night long, your body has been at work while you have been sleeping. During this cycle it has been absorbing and using the foods eaten during the previous day. This is also the time when the body heals and repairs itself from the exertion and stress on the muscles and entire body. By morning the body goes into releasing and eliminating waste products. Elimination is the window from 4:00 a.m. to 12:00 noon.

When you rise in the morning, you have essentially been fasting all night. You have not had food since you went to bed. Your blood sugar is now starting to drop. Getting your blood sugar back up is the first order of business. When your feet hit the floor, your first priority is to break your fast. Breakfast!

Low-glycemic fruit is going to bring up your blood sugar without causing an insulin response or spike. Most low-glycemic fruit, such as apples and pears, are harder to chew. If you can remember *The Harder to Chew, the More You Lose!* you will subconsciously choose low- glycemic fruits. Especially in Phase 1, the fruits we prefer are the watery fruits. Watery fruits help us to flush and to cleanse the body. We call fruits "nature's scrub brush." Fruits for breakfast will facilitate elimination because of the watery quality, the fiber, and the quick digestion time. They will also help to improve the health of your colon and your liver.

Have a nice big bowl of fruit. Have as much as you want. It is going to help with elimination all morning. Remember that low-glycemic fruit digests and leaves the stomach in twenty minutes. It is going to go through your small intestines where nutrition is absorbed. Then it goes into the colon, moving things along. FYF4Good mandates a second serving of fruit in the afternoon or evening (following the proper food combining rules). The more fruit you eat, the more you are going to lose. In the summer months, when so many delicious fruits are available and in season, you can have more than two servings of fruit per day. Listen to your brain. If you want more, eat it. You might be hungry for it because you need to replenish important vitamins and nutrients found in the fresh fruits, such as vitamin C, vitamin A, etc. Cherries contain serotonin, as does kiwi, and are great before bedtime as a snack. It helps you to have a good sleep. Fruits and vegetables are so important on FYF4Good. Please refer to the section "Selecting Fruits and Vegetables" in chapter eleven.

FISH
What Fish Should We Avoid, And Which Are Best for Us?

FYF4Good recommends avoiding any type of shellfish or any other scavenger fish. Shellfish are fatty fish and contain neurotoxins in their livers, resulting from what they have been exposed to. Pregnant women are advised not to eat shellfish at all during the pregnancy because of the high level of potential neurotoxins they contain. Additionally, avoid any fish (or food for that matter) from China. The tilapia, for example, that comes from China has been shown to be raised in waste water. You can bet that this fish contains high levels of toxins. Avoid tilapia from any country; it has a cheap, low-nutrient value and is potentially a very unsafe fish to eat.

Some people really enjoy lobster on a special occasion. If you want lobster once or twice a year, it is not going to kill you, but do not eat surf and turf (fish with red meat). They digest differently so you do not want them in your stomach at the same time. They will really be difficult to break down and digest. It is very high in fat and will give your liver/gallbladder a workout! You will pay for it!

Wild Salmon and Other Healthy Wild Fish

Salmon is one of the best choices. It is really tasty and is a great source for omega-3 fatty acids. Salmon is one of the only fish rich in vitamin B12. It is great for the brain as it contains DHA. In a three-ounce serving you can get five hundred to one thousand milligrams of all the combined omega-3 fatty acids. Eat only wild salmon, and absolutely avoid farm-raised salmon. Farmed salmon are not fed what wild salmon eat normally in nature. They are fed processed feed. Also, because it is a very fatty fish rich in the omega-3 fatty acids, the risk of ingesting mercury is very high. The toxins will be stored in the fat … like they are in humans!

Notice the color of the wild salmon. If it is a deep bright beautiful orange color, this would be the best pick. Farmed salmon is a faded orange color. But food colorings may have been added to make them look darker, so be careful where you buy your fish. Canned wild salmon is also great to eat and keep on hand in the pantry.

When eating fatty fish like salmon, it is a good idea to eat some fresh cilantro. Cilantro has been known to help cleanse the body and chelate the toxic metals that are often stored in fatty fish. Take a bunch of organic cilantro and put it into a food processor or chop finely. Add two to three cloves of minced fresh garlic, juice of one or two lemons, Pink Himalayan Salt, and pepper. Then you have delicious cilantro dressing for your salmon! Cilantro is also an incredible source of antioxidants so always have some on hand.

Some great types of wild fish to eat with high omega-3 fatty acids are wild Atlantic or Spanish mackerel, freshwater Coho salmon or wild salmon from Alaska, trout, Pacific halibut, and Pacific sardines (canned). Deep-sea fish have the most fat and are rich in the omega-3 fatty acids so these are also great choices. Exercise extreme caution when eating fish such as sushi, sashimi, or any kind of raw or undercooked fish, as there is a higher risk than ever of ingesting parasites carried by the fish. This is predominantly due to large quantities of fish imported from China and other Asian countries. Do you know the source, and is it safe?

CRANFLUSH

And of course, last but not least, we cannot forget our CranFlush! CranFlush is a required staple. You must drink eighty-one ounces per day. This is three large glass Voss bottles filled eighty percent with water, then adding unsweetened not from concentrate 100 percent cranberry juice to the top. For CranGingerFlush, add one teaspoon to one tablespoon of freshly juiced ginger root.

CHAPTER TEN

TROUBLESHOOTING FOR GOOD RESULTS

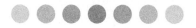

When following the FYF4Good Lifestyle, you will begin eating, maybe for the first time in your life, the way God intended. Healthy foods, proper nutrition, correct food combining. Your body will start changing immediately. Sometimes you will see or feel the changes, other times the changes may not be obvious to you, but know they are happening. Patience is everything. This section includes some of the most common questions from Buddies on this Lifestyle, what you need to watch out for, and what not to worry about when we are on the road to optimal health.

SUGAR CRAVINGS

Life is so SWEET without the Sugar

It all started so gradually and innocently, I never felt it coming. I never saw any warning signs or felt that I was in danger—but I was! I had an addiction, or rather, it had me. If we really understood the seriousness of this, we would fight to eliminate it—but we can't. We're hooked. And it's only getting worse.

It was a celebration party, a holiday, a reward. It was comfort when hurting. It was a snack to hold me over until dinner. My earliest memories include sugar as an occasional treat. It was a part of family holidays, birthdays, parties at school, Thanksgiving, Christmas, basically any time we were celebrating or happy about something. A few nights a week we had dessert after dinner, but only if we cleaned our plates.

Grandma made *the best* cakes and pies for every family birthday and special holiday. People used to get out of line at potlucks to go to the dessert table and get Grandma's pie before it was gone! Her fudge and peanut brittle at Christmas were worth the eleven and one half month wait. And Mom's homemade ice cream was *amazing!* I couldn't get enough!!

When I finally moved out on my own, I was FREE! Free to eat what I wanted and when I wanted. Sounds awesome! Looking back, it was a recipe for disaster. Ice cream every night. Fast food often. Grilled cheese, chips, dips, French fries, hamburgers on white bread buns—they all became my friends! And the soft drinks, *lots* of Coke Classic. I started hearing that fast food wasn't good to eat, but I wasn't feeling bad. It must just affect *SOME* people. Surely not me!

Fast forward to April 2015, and I am starting FYF4Good. I have been pouring so much sugar into my body that I am now addicted, and I am *certain* that, for the next year, I am going to have to painfully deny myself all sugar, every day, as I struggle to lose the 100 pounds of extra fat I have gained. But I am determined to get the fat off.

What I found was, after about two weeks of focusing on learning this Lifestyle, I was no longer craving the sugar. In fact, as time has gone on, I am tempted less and less as my paradigm is shifting and my body and mind are adjusting. I am getting healthier, my body is getting used to no processed sugars, and I am feeling so much better!! I am thinking more clearly, sleeping more deeply, my hormones are balanced, aches and pains are less, it's no wonder I have become a nicer person! This truly is a *Lifestyle for a Lifetime!* And life is *Much Sweeter* without the sugar!

~*FYF4Good Coach Jennifer*

We met for the First Time on FYF4Good

I never knew my sister Jennifer. Oh we have the same parents, grew up in the same house, have spent at least one holiday together every year of our adult lives, but I never knew my sister. You see my sister and I were like oil and water. Oh there were obvious differences (I was twenty-two months younger than her, six inches taller, had dark brown hair (vs. her blond hair) and listened to Led Zeppelin and Lynyrd Skynyrd; she liked Chicago, James Taylor and the Carpenters) but that wasn't it. I thought she didn't like me, an obnoxious little sister wanting to tag along. But that wasn't it at all. (Okay, maybe that had a little to do with it.)

I never knew my sister Jennifer. We really met for the first time about three months after she started the FYF4Good Lifestyle. She called to tell me what she was doing. I did not recognize the person on the other end of the phone. Her voice had energy, and she talked with such excitement. She sounded happy! And she wanted to share something about her life with me. How could this possibly be the same person I grew up with?

After spending more than two years living the FYF4Good Lifestyle, I now understand. My sister was so addicted to sugar. The sugar not only put fat onto her body, but it made her depressed and unhappy. She was always irritated or angry with me. And she definitely did not like me.

I never knew my sister Jennifer, until that day she called. The sugar was gone, the fat was rapidly burning off her body, her hormones were balancing, and she was happy—I think for the first time in her life. Now we talk almost every day on the phone, we have traveled together, and I consider her a close friend. Who would have ever thought, life could be so-so-so sweet without the sugar.

~ *FYF4Good Coach Kathleen*

Sugar cravings will disappear, on average, in about two weeks after starting Phase 1. The trick to getting rid of these cravings is first to eliminate sugar, flour, and starch from your Lifestyle. If you were eating a lot of sugar and were a sugar-aholic, you know that sugar is addictive and is similar to cocaine on the brain... sometimes as strong as an opiate addiction. For some it can be very painful and there could be symptoms of fatigue, headache, sleeplessness and muscle aches.

It is important to eat extra protein during this time. Have at least two to three good protein meals a day. Jackie's Chicken Salad is the best choice for you right now. Have a big bowl in the refrigerator, along with your arugula and kale. When you get sugar cravings, eat more Jackie's Chicken Salad. Have it multiple times a day if you need it. Make sure you also have your daily goat yogurt with nuts, and the two servings of fruit. Drink, drink, drink the CranFlush to get yourself flushed, cleansed, hydrated, and provide your body with the phytonutrients, antioxidants and anti-inflammatory benefits. These cravings should resolve if you immediately eat some protein. Fatigue, headaches, sleeplessness and muscle aches are all symptoms of the sugar detoxification or your blood sugar trying to stay consistent and stable. Hang in there! If you are following this *Lifestyle to a "T"* in a few weeks your body makes the switch to burn your fat for energy. When this happens the symptoms should disappear!

One cute little trick Jackie uses, if you are tempted with a sugary treat or bread, pick it up and smell it. Take a good, deep whiff. It is weird how it works, but it does. Take for example licorice. There is no taste to licorice. It is the aroma of the licorice that tells the brain what it is. Many love it and many hate it. But if you pinch your nose and chew the licorice, you will find that it has no taste. You will be satisfied with just smelling a tempting food and you will have the power to walk away.

MEDICAL CONDITIONS AND MEDICATIONS

Caution: *Please consult your health care practitioner to titrate your medications. FYF4Good does NOT recommend you increase or decrease your medications on your own.*

We cannot stress this enough, so we will say it again here. If you have any serious medical issues such as a recent heart attack, kidney disease, or liver disease, it is not advisable to begin FYF4Good until you consult with your health care practitioner. If you have medical conditions that require you to take medications, or you are pregnant or are breast feeding a baby that is less than six months old, it is recommended that you review FYF4Good with your health care practitioner and get their approval before beginning. If you have had a gastric bypass or weight-loss surgery, again it is highly recommended that you review this Lifestyle together with your health care practitioner. This is a great way to have them on your team to help with managing your health. You will be the winner from this arrangement because this information can be added to your medical chart, and many questions you have due to changes you experience may be answered on the phone, often without going in for an appointment. This can be especially true and crucial with titration and management of medications. The body becomes very dependent on the medications, so they must be titrated by a trained medical professional.

Keep in mind there are side effects from medications (blood pressure, blood sugar, and thyroid medications may cause strange side effects) especially when your body is improving. If you start becoming light-headed, dizzy, weak, tired, feel a need to lie down, have extremely low blood pressure (hypotension), or you feel like fainting, call and see your health care practitioner immediately. It may be as simple as needing your medications adjusted since your body is getting healthier and the body is very sensitive to the dosages of the medications. Knowledge is power. Ignorance breeds fear and can be very dangerous. "The doctor who treats himself, has a fool for a patient."

PROBLEMS RELATED TO SEVERE OVERFAT

If you are severely overfat, keep in mind that you almost certainly have a hormone imbalance that causes chaos in your body. This is a physiological fact. Your liver will take up the burden to detoxify and help your body return to normal hormonal function. You should assume you will have liver congestion from the excess fat. You will have more plateaus as well when you have chosen the Lifestyle, since your body must make changes related to the loss of your fat. Make sure you drink plenty of CranFlush and that you are following this *Lifestyle to a "T"* and eating appropriately. Make certain you are eating goat yogurt with nuts every day. It helps the colon. As soon as the colon is working properly, it will reduce the stress on the liver. Anything that helps the colon helps the liver.

It makes sense there will be constipation issues until you get your hormones under control and your gastrointestinal (GI) track moving again. Remember peristalsis is the wave-like motion that moves food from the esophagus through to the rectum: mouth to anus. If you are severely over-fat chances are pretty good that this is not functioning properly, but the good news is that it will come back. Stay the course, and every day your body will be getting healthier.

You are not in this alone. Many large people with a lot of fat to lose, have found success with FYF4Good. For more details refer to chapter seven: "FYF4Good Power100 Heroes" or visit FlushYourFat4Good.com. If your goal is to lose a lot of fat quickly and to get on track for optimal health take advantage of our live support calls. Also do not forget to join the Flush Your Fat 4Good "Buddies" Facebook Group for extra support. Pillar #8: Support & Accountability (described in chapter two) is one of the most important Pillars for Power100 Heroes. This is a major Paradigm Shift. The support calls will help you make the shift into a new way of thinking about your relationship with food.

It is important for all of us to understand that if we know that certain foods are not good for us, but we eat them anyway, that is an abusive situation. We call this *Stockholm Food Syndrome*— being in love with foods that will harm you. How many times have you said or heard someone say, "I know I shouldn't eat that but I'm going to do it anyway"? Think about that. You know that certain food will be harmful in so many ways, but the choice is still to eat it. That is not only addiction to an abuser but thinking that you may never have access to that food again. Like being in love with an abusive boyfriend or girlfriend and afraid you will never meet another companion again. The new Paradigm Shift is of one saying, "I know I shouldn't eat that so therefore I'm not going to!" Now there's no guilt or regrets and pride starts to develop about your new found control over your own life with respect. FYF4Good teaches our Power100 Heroes about the foods that will help them heal, feel great and assist them in burning off the fat. This is helping them to have a new relationship and appreciation for their body and the foods that are meant for optimal health and well-being. Everyone can benefit from this new way of thinking.

Check out our website, FlushYourFat4Good.com to learn how to join the live support calls. It is great to listen, learn and ask. On our website you can also get access to the support call library. You can also listen to these archived calls at your leisure. Our hearts run deep for our Power100

Heroes as we so admire them for giving life another chance. We love helping EVERYONE, reach your goals.

NOT FEELING HUNGRY?

This is very common for people when they first start on FYF4Good. Your body needs a lot of protein and healthy vitamins and minerals to function correctly. If you are struggling to follow the Lifestyle because you are not hungry, ask yourself, "How many bowel movements am I having each day?" This may be a strange question to ask yourself, but if the answer is not two to three, then you may be constipated. Why? Because if your bowels have not emptied completely every day, it can be assumed that elimination is not what is considered normal. Three to four bowel movements a day is ideal. If your bowels are not moving and evacuating the stool, you could feel backed up or bloated. This means your digestive tract will be sluggish, your metabolic rate is lower, and therefore you can experience less hunger. The faster the metabolic rate, the more bowel movements you will have, and the hungrier you will be.

Being hungry is a good thing. Your food has been digested, assimilated and eliminated from your intestines, so now your body is telling you it is ready for more nutrients. Bowel movements are extremely important for optimal health and fat loss. Also keep in mind that 70 to 80 percent of your immune system is in your gut. Optimal digestion allows nutrients to be absorbed for energy, health, and burning of fat to ultimately be eliminated. Stay the course, and most importantly, make sure you are getting your two servings of low-glycemic fruit each day, you are drinking eighty-one ounces of CranFlush, and eating crunchy vegetables with your protein. It takes time to get the digestive system working optimally so don't get discouraged. Keep eating!

In addition, when starting, many people are not hungry because their digestive system and metabolism are functioning on a very low level from years of yo-yo dieting, calorie counting, starving, and portion control. These are the people who may be at risk of gaining a large amount of weight in a very short time. The body initially wants to conserve everything it can because food has been restricted in the past. Keep eating according to the FYF4Good recommendations. Your body needs to learn that your lifestyle has changed, and since food and nutrients will not be restricted, there will be better digestion and absorption. We at FYF4Good get very excited when we hear of Buddies bowel movements improving and increasing to two to three maybe even four bowel movements a day. It may take your body a little time to get there, but it will happen. Keep eating!

FYF4Good is different because you are going to be **eating** yourself lean. For this Lifestyle to work best, it is advised that you do not ever get to the point where you are super hungry or famished. Some people tell us that they have a hard time eating so much. They say they are okay with eating something but not very much. You do not have to eat a full meal or full serving— just eat a small amount to trigger digestion. We want you to listen to your brain. You want to "stoke" the fire which revs up the metabolism, ideally by not going much longer than four hours after eating protein. We want to keep our blood sugars from dropping dramatically by eating something as soon as the food has digested and left the stomach.

Up until now, your metabolism has been slowed, and it probably still is, until your brain learns that you are going to supply consistent "fuel" in the tank. When the brain does not detect the fuel (food), the metabolism will slow, and the body will begin to retain the fat. When the brain detects there is a steady supply of fuel, that digestion is occurring, and blood sugars stay consistent, then the fat is burned, and the metabolism increases to higher levels.

In the first couple of weeks, water weight comes off from the elimination of bloat and edema in the interstitial tissues. To keep the metabolism fired up, practice *The 5 P's: Proper Planning Prevents Poor Performance!*

CONSTIPATION

"Normal bowel movements" is defined medically as one to three or four bowel movements per day, according to Cecil's *Textbook of Medicine*. Therefore, if you have fewer than three stools per week, you are experiencing constipation. One stool per week is considered severe constipation. One of the most important goals of the FYF4Good Lifestyle is to restore normal bowel function. If you are constipated, do not feel bad about it. Believe it or not, most people are, but do not realize it! Many people will say they are not constipated because they have a bowel movement every other day. No, this is considered constipation! As a precaution, should you have unusual, sudden or severe issues associated with the bowels or constipation, it is recommended to see your health care practitioner to rule out any serious medical problems associated with it. Other than severe issues, if you are experiencing constipation what are some things you can do about this?

- Are you remembering to take your digestive enzymes?
- Are you eating goat yogurt with nuts every day?
- Are you taking your probiotic before bed (right before brushing your teeth)?
- Are you eating enough fruit? Twice a day?
- Are you drinking eighty-one ounces of CranFlush through the day?

If the answer is yes to any of these questions, try doubling up on them for a few days until everything gets started again. If the answer is no, what are you thinking? Following this *Lifestyle to a "T"* is essential. This is *Health by Design, Not by Default!* So let's get going! Many times we hear of a Buddy saying they have never had constipation issues before. However, they have been overfat for years. Therefore, the joy for us is to tell them, "The Lifestyle is working!" You are losing fat! However, there are toxins in the fat, and when fat is burned, these fat cells and toxins will filter through the liver. Any time that you see bowel problems in a person who is not eliminating waste at least two or three times a day, you most likely have a congested or a compromised liver. The liver is said to have over five hundred vital functions, but one of the primary jobs is to detoxify the colon. After a lifetime of being overfat and obese you have a 30 to 90 percent chance of developing a "fatty liver," also known as Non-Alcoholic Fatty Liver Disease or NAFLD. Eating and living this *Lifestyle to a "T"* will help take the burden off your liver to also aid the liver to cleanse, restore optimal function, and rejuvenate. So it makes physiological sense to look at the liver when you are constipated.

Ways to Aid Liver Function and Restore Elimination

How do we cleanse the liver? CranFlush, CranFlush, CranFlush. Drink at least eighty-one ounces of CranFlush every day. Make sure you are eating at least two large servings of low-glycemic fruit every day. And do not forget the goat yogurt with nuts. If you are still "NOT HUNGRY" or still "CONSTIPATED," five OPTIONS to try would be:

- Jackie's Jump Start (first forty-eight hours (two days) of fruit, yogurt with nuts, organic coffee and recommended milk, at least eighty-one ounces of CranFlush and of course all of the recommended FYF4Good supplements). The next forty-eight hours, the same but add Jackie's Turkey Soup. And then the last two days, all the same but add Jackie's Chicken Salad. Keep reading for details!
- Make sure you are getting at least eighty-one ounces of CranFlush. Add a little fresh ginger juice since our delicious CranGingerFlush is amazing.
- Squeeze half of a lemon into four to six ounces of hot water and drink it first thing in the morning before your fruit and one hour before bedtime to help with clearing fat out of the liver.
- If constipation is severe, you may want to see your health care practitioner. You may also check the recommendations on FlushYourFat4Good.com.
- Be patient, as it will gradually improve. It is pretty much a "common textbook case" to see this from time to time.

There are three stages of constipation you may experience on your FYF4Good journey.

Constipation Occurring Early in FYF4Good Phase 1

Early Constipation may occur during the first one to three weeks on Phase 1 for some people. If you are following the *Lifestyle to a "T"* you have just put your body into "Nutritional Ketosis"—what is called an accelerated fat-burning state! This means the fat is starting to melt away, and the toxins that were being stored in the fat are now flowing into the liver. The liver may become congested and sluggish. This may cause gas, cramping, and nausea. And do not forget, like many of us "sugar-aholics," we have developed a fatty liver from simply being overweight or eating too much sugar, similar to that of someone who drinks a lot of alcohol.

Therefore, if this happens to you, then you CANNOT expect to be regular! Your digestion simply may not be working optimally. You most likely have not had correct functioning of your peristalsis for years. You may have when you were a child, but the vast majority of FYF4Good Buddies were not digesting well until this current Lifestyle.

Constipation Occurring During a Phase 1 Plateau

Another issue with constipation may occur when you have plateaued for a month or two. You have been on the *Lifestyle to a "T"* for a while, experienced fat loss, are still following what you should to a "T" but are constipated. You are probably losing more fat with toxins in this stage. This is especially true if you have had a very bad diet or have used a lot of drugs (legal or recreationally) over the years. Additionally, fat will sometimes clog up the liver and this is where the five options previously mentioned will come in to play, especially Jackie's Jump Start.

Keep in mind, you lose fat in stages. Your body has got to get used to your new body, adjust to its new size and be able to function appropriately. You have to slow down to make the turn and your body knows that.

Constipation Occurring after Several Months on FYF-4Good Phase 1

You have had great results from following the Phase 1 Lifestyle for many months, but now you are constipated. Take a look at what you are eating. Are you eating fewer fruits and vegetables? Are you getting enough Cran-Flush? Are you eating a serving of goat yogurt with nuts every day? Go through the details of your day. If you still think you are doing everything right, your body might be working through losing the visceral fat. This will cause your liver to be congested from the fat and toxins. Add an extra serving of fruit in the evening. Since fruit passes through the stomach quickly, it will go through your colon during the night and push the poop through.

There are additional things you can do to help constipation.

First, analyze your day to make sure you really are following this *Lifestyle to a "T"*: ALL 8 ESSENTIAL PILLARS! If the answer is yes, then go back to the basics for seventy-two hours. No experimenting with recipes. No cheese. No extra seasonings. Make it SIMPLE. Jackie's Jump Start is to consume low-glycemic fruits and vegetables, Jackie's Chicken Salad, Jackie's Turkey Soup, goat yogurt with nuts, organic coffee and recommended milk, and of course your supplements.

Always remember to take your RECOMMENDED supplements. If you have tried to cut corners and are taking a synthetic supplement, STOP! These can create constipation as well. The good news is, it will all improve as you continue to eat this Lifestyle way.

Jackie's Six-Day Jump Start

If you have severe constipation, follow these steps of Jackie's Six-Day Jump Start:

> *Days one and two*: Eat only fruit, yogurt with nuts, CranFlush, supplements, and your FYF4Good Latte following the proper food combining rules.
>
> *Days three and four*: Eat fruit, yogurt with nuts, Jackie's Turkey Soup, CranFlush, supplements and your FYF4Good Latte.
>
> *Days five and six*: Eat fruit, yogurt with nuts, Jackie's Turkey Soup, Jackie's Chicken Salad, CranFlush, supplements, and your FYF-4Good Latte.

This jump start of six days will allow you to have all the nutrition you need but will keep the burden of digestion down to a minimum so that these foods will be allowed to go through easily.

Double-up on your digestive enzymes before each protein meal and your probiotic before you go to bed. Should you need a colon health supplement (please see FlushYourFat4Good.com for a recommendation), take it one hour before bed, then follow with the probiotic, and brush your teeth and go to bed. As you are sleeping, they both will be working throughout the entire digestive system to improve elimination. Eating simple meals and providing the extra supplements gives your body a break to start functioning again.

The goal is to get the digestive tract working with digestion, absorption, and elimination as it did before we became toxic and overfat. Hippocrates said, "Let your food be your medicine and your medicine be your food." FYF4Good recommends eating foods to utilize the healing powers of the food to help you achieve health. We discourage the use of prescription or over-the-counter digestive aids taken on a regular basis. Taking these means the digestive system is not functioning as it should, and these could inhibit your ability to lose fat and achieve optimal health. The exception of course is if you are under the care of a health care practitioner. Ultimately, you can work with your health care practitioner to eventually get off any digestive aids when digestion and elimination improve.

You can also try increasing your coffee intake, but always make sure you drink organic coffee. FYF4Good recommends drinking one to three cups of coffee each day. Coffee helps to get the bowels moving. It works as a diuretic and perks up metabolism. It is also rich in antioxidants. Coffee helps your mood, increases your intelligence, and has been shown to prevent certain cancers. So, you might want to do a little more coffee to get those bowels moving. If you do not want the jitters that some people may get, drink organic dark roast coffee! Lighter roasted coffees have more caffeine, and pesticides may be the cause of nausea and jitters, so always choose organic coffee.

Regardless, do NOT be alarmed! Again, fat is lost in stages. When you are losing fat, no matter how long you have been on FYF4Good, some people occasionally become constipated. Get together with your Coach, get into the Facebook Group, or get on our live weekly support calls to reach out for help. Most often, a little troubleshooting and fine-tuning will get you back in sync. It is best to make sure you practice the 8th Pillar, Support & Accountability. Stay in contact by text, phone, email, or private message through the Facebook Group, with your Coach and/or Buddy. This is the key to great success. In order to win, you must participate.

DIARRHEA

The FYF4Good Lifestyle should not cause diarrhea, although diarrhea can be a sign of detoxifying. If you have a yeast overgrowth in your body, you will frequently experience loose stools when the yeast "dies off" and is eliminated in what is called a "Herxheimer Reaction." (In chapter two refer to "Pillar #5: Detoxing" for more information.) You can also get diarrhea from certain fruits, but this is rare. Sometimes the naturally occurring sorbitol in an apple, for example, may initiate loose stools, especially if you have eaten a very large (or more than one) apple. If for any reason you have diarrhea for a long period of time, consult with your health care practitioner. You can get dehydrated quickly. It may be an indicator of another, more serious issue, and you want to get a timely diagnosis.

YEAST OVERGROWTH

We all have yeast in our bodies, but when there is overgrowth, it can become a very common yeast infection called *candidiasis*. When a pregnant woman delivers vaginally, she can pass this yeast to the baby during delivery because the yeast fungus called *Candida* is a naturally occurring microorganism in the vaginal tract. For a baby, thrush (a coated tongue), diaper rash, cradle cap (fungal red rash on head) often indicates a yeast infection from this fungus family and is very common. The baby's immune system is not developed to produce antibodies until about six months of age and not fully developed until about five years of age, so the baby might have a difficult time initially fighting off the overgrowth. This is why it is important to wash your hands before touching a newborn baby. Breastfeeding mothers must be careful and diligent to eat properly and get enough rest. As long as the mother takes care of herself, and works with a pediatrician, in the vast majority of cases, the baby will reverse the overgrowth symptoms and recover beautifully.

Adults who have had a lot of stress with a challenged immune function, have frequently taken antibiotics and certain medications, or have eaten poorly for many years such as too many sodas, cow dairy products, sugar, starches, vinegars, donuts, chips, cookies, and crackers, etc., may have caused the development of an overgrowth of yeast in their bodies. Years of NOT eating FRESH foods can cause high-insulin secretion in the blood, insulin resistance, and obesity (with twenty or more pounds to lose). Low protein consumption and even starving yourself at times, will also contribute to setting your body up to have a minor or major infection of systemic yeast overgrowth.

With yeast overgrowth, you may bloat and look puffy. Toenail and skin fungus are the most common minor forms of *Candidiasis*. Brain fog, severe fatigue, allergies, gas and bloating are also common symptoms of what may be a more serious extensive yeast infection that can circulate through the blood and into the organs. Dysbiosis leads to "leaky gut" as an example, develops when there is damage to the walls of the gut causing a host of problems including severe malabsorption. After birth, we gradually and naturally accumulate yeast microorganisms, so we all will have some yeast in our bodies. When our immune system is functioning optimally, along with a healthy eating and lifestyle, the combination helps our body to work hard to keep it at bay.

The immune system is compromised by the yeast overgrowth. When the immune system is functioning below 50 percent, the yeast infection may start to significantly take over. Supporting your immune system is imperative. It will allow the body to kill the yeast. Because there is no starch, no sugar, excellent nutritional supplements, and the consistent flushing with fluids recommended in FYF4Good Phase 1, this is the best possible way to get a handle on controlling yeast issues.

But be aware, if you do have a yeast issue, once you start to incorporate the FYF4Good Lifestyle, and follow ALL of the 8 Essential Pillars, especially the first six, you may physically experience yeast die-off called a Herxheimer Reaction. As the overgrowth of yeast that has been harboring in your gut or even in your blood stream starts to "die off," toxins are released. Some of the symptoms as previously mentioned may include rashes in large or small areas on the skin, white coating on the tongue, brain fog, feeling terrible, fatigue, irritation in the nasal passages or mouth, or even in the lungs, and stomach aches or nausea. If you have an insulin spike from increased blood sugar in the blood stream, that sugar will feed the yeast. Conversely, if you do not eat, and your blood sugar drops, the yeast will also proliferate, which is another reason why skipping meals is not recommended.

RIDE THIS OUT! Within three days on FYF4Good, most people will start to feel better. We all have yeast in our guts. It is a naturally occurring microorganism. But when we do not eat right and are consuming starches (bread, rice, potatoes, crackers, etc.), vinegars, and sugars, or are on rounds of antibiotics or certain medications, the yeast can act up and grow again. Keep in mind if you have to go on another antibiotic, eat your yogurt at least two to three hours before or after taking your antibiotic. Same thing with taking your probiotic at night time. You do not want the antibiotic to kill the good probiotics in your yogurt. They will be extremely helpful to you while on the antibiotic. **What you are eating is 95 percent of the solution!** Stay the course.

NAUSEA

Remember, the liver detoxes the body. It filters all the excess hormones. Some people, when they first start FYF4Good, may feel a little nausea because their hormones are completely out of balance. As the hormones start to normalize, the excess hormones are taken up and processed in the liver. In addition, those who have chronically eaten large quantities of sugar, may experience withdrawal symptoms, one of which may be nausea.

Make sure you are drinking the CranFlush. Make sure you are taking all the recommended supplements. They are recommended for good reasons to achieve rapid fat loss while supporting bodily functions. DO NOT ever substitute "cheap" synthetic supplements.

Of course, you can also feel nausea if you are fighting a cold or flu bug or some other ailment, or are dehydrated. Stay hydrated.

Phytates

Another reason you are nauseous or you have a stomach ache may be due to eating unsoaked nuts. Raw nuts and seeds must be soaked before eating: Soak them overnight in water with one tablespoon Pink Himalayan Salt or Sea Salt; rinse thoroughly and heat in a low oven (170 degrees Fahrenheit) or dehydrator only until they are dried. If you do not soak the nuts, they will contain phytates. Phytates are there to keep the nut dormant until the proper minerals, moisture, and heat are applied to bring the nut to life.

Phytates are anti-nutrients or plant toxins. They are found in numerous foods, including wheat, barley, rice, beans, nuts, legumes, seeds, and soy, and are consumed in small amounts by everyone. Most phytates are dissolved by the digestive system. However, if too much is consumed, phytic acid can bind minerals in the gut before they are absorbed, and it can wreak havoc with our digestive enzymes. Phytates directly reduce the digestibility of starches, proteins, and fats. If you have ever eaten nuts and find stomach discomfort or nausea after eating the un-soaked nuts, the phytates could be the culprit.

When eating nuts on a regular basis, as we do in FYF4Good, it is important that you soak them properly to remove the phytates. Nuts that have been soaked are also softer and easier to digest. They provide a source of live protein and nutrients, and they have wonderful healing oils in them.

Nuts are really seeds. If you look in nature, nuts fall to the ground into the dirt in their shells. Rain decomposes the shells, and they fall off. The nuts are left, and as more rain falls, the minerals in the dirt, along with the water and the heat from the sun, remove the phytates, activating the nut (seed). The seed is now live and begins to sprout, take root, and grow in the soil. The live seed activates the powerhouse of enzymes and properties for the seed to germinate and grow to a mature plant. Consuming this live powerhouse is a benefit to the body.

ALLERGIES

If you "think" you are allergic to something, see your health care practitioner to get properly diagnosed. A rash from a yeast "die-off" is not an allergy. Hives and rashes may be toxins coming out through the skin near the site where they were being stored. The largest organ of elimination in the body is the skin. (In chapter two refer to "Pillar #5: Detoxing" for more information.)

Maybe you feel like you cannot breathe or your sinuses are clogged. Look first at your environment. Is it spring? Is there a lot of pollen in the air? Or is there a construction site nearby with a lot of dust? Are you going through a yeast "die-off"? Are you getting sick? Often the excessive mucous in the sinus cavities will release and drain along with mucous in other areas such as the lungs or colon, as you are cleansing your body. You can also clean out your sinuses with an OTC (over the counter) NeilMed Sinus Rinse. Many times nausea comes from the sinuses. Let it run its course. If you have concern, consult your health care practitioner.

Some people have claimed that they are allergic to CranFlush. They feel the taste is too tart. Understandably, if you have never tasted it before, it is going to taste different or unusual. CranFlush is the best way possible to cleanse, detox, and flush your liver, kidneys, and bladder, and the benefits and nutritional properties (vitamins K, C, E, manganese, riboflavin, potassium, magnesium) of cranberries are tremendous. Cranberries are very beneficial for almost everyone.

Did you know that cranberries may reduce the risk of urinary tract infections? They help in the prevention of certain types of cancer, help to improve the immune system, have anti-inflammatory and antioxidant effects, and help to decrease blood pressure. Cranberries are considered one of the world's healthiest foods. If you are having difficulty getting the CranFlush down initially, you can dilute it with more water than we recommend. FYF4Good mandates the minimum recommended quantity of CranFlush every day. This is the best natural way to flush out the fat and toxins from your body and keep it cleansed through Phase 1. Believe it or not, after a bit of time you will learn to love it and you will crave the CranFlush!

Most people with food allergies have been diagnosed and already know what they are allergic to. For example, if you know you are allergic to soy milk, you can substitute goat, hemp, or flax milk. Vegans who follow the FYF4Good Lifestyle eat soy yogurt instead of goat yogurt. They make it themselves because it is difficult to find unsweetened soy yogurt. Vegans can also make yogurt out of hemp and flax milk. If you look at the cultures that eat soy on a regular basis, for example the Japanese, there are groups of people that live well into the triple digits with very little incidence of breast or other cancers. These people typically die of old age.

If you continue to have a concern, see the studies on the FYF4Good website regarding the safety of soy or talk to your health care practitioner. Knowledge is power. And take a copy of FYF4Good with you so your health care practitioner can review what you are doing.

EXTREME FATIGUE

If this happens during the first few weeks on FYF4Good, congratulations! You may be having your DAY OF EXHAUSTION (D.O.E.). This can occur anytime during the first few weeks but may also happen again. Initially, it just means that your brain is making the conversion to burning your stored fat for fuel rather than glucose from starches, sugars, and/or other foods you have eaten. This is what we want. This means your brain has made the transition, and you will be burning the premium fuel for energy.

This is like burning the highest-octane fuel possible for energy, and energy is what you should receive from this transition. The fatigue will go away and will be replaced with a sustained burst of vitality, energy, and a tremendous sense of well-being. After your DOE, you might also notice better sleep.

If you have been on the Lifestyle awhile, or if this is lasting more than a few days, first make sure you are drinking three bottles minimum of your CranFlush and are not dehydrated. Dehydration can cause extreme fatigue, but here are a few more considerations that could be in play:

Are you taking the recommended digestive enzymes with your protein meals?

If not, why not? Without digestive enzymes you cannot absorb minerals, iron, or protein. Remember, we need to supplement our body with digestive enzymes because most of us, especially if we are carrying excess fat, do not have enough enzymes in our digestive tracts to properly digest our food. (If you forget to take digestive enzymes before your meal, take them as soon as you remember, during or after.) As we age, we lose 15 percent of these digestive enzymes every ten years.

Are you eating enough protein?

If you are not getting in at least two good protein meals a day, in addition to your goat yogurt with nuts, and your soy, goat, hemp, or flax milk in your organic coffee, then you are not eating enough protein. This can make you tired. It can also cause you to wake up in the middle of the night hungry or craving sugar. Protein is the building block for your muscles, and if we do not get enough, our body will tell us. Protein is the fuel propelling the fat burning. Most people do not eat nearly enough protein and almost every function in the body depends on proteins. Protein consumption is necessary to have beautiful skin. The body breaks down the protein to amino acids and sends the appropriate amino acids to the skin. Our skin utilizes protein to look young and healthy. And as we shrink in size, the amino acid building blocks from the protein we eat will help rejuvenate, repair, and regenerate the skin, and shrink it in a healthy way rendering better elasticity. *Bottom line*: Make sure you are getting plenty of protein throughout the day.

Are you getting sick?

We are not immune to sickness just because we are now eating and supplementing our bodies. The body may occasionally become infected with bacteria, a cold, or the flu. This is the natural cycle of building our immune system.

Lack of digestive enzymes, too little protein, not getting enough sleep, stress, and coming down with a cold are the most common reasons for feeling tired. With all of the great fresh whole foods and nutrifying with pure supplements in the FYF4Good Lifestyle, energy should increase to a level that most of us have not experienced in a very long time.

MOUTH SORES

Daily we eat a lot of fruits and vegetables. Buy organic when possible. If you eat out a lot, the restaurants may buy produce that is loaded with pesticides. This can be overwhelming on the body, and these toxins may be released by the mucous membranes in the mouth and you may experience burning. Luckily, the mucus membranes in the mouth are very quick to heal.

Do not be fooled into thinking CranFlush is causing the outbreak. There is a cleansing of the mucous membranes taking place. Try diluting the CranFlush as much as it takes to make it tolerable, but do not stop drinking it as it will help speed-up the process of flushing and cleansing the toxins out of the tissues. Cranberries are often used to help soothe sores in the mouth.

Try to minimize the irritation to the area until the sores go away. As always, if you are concerned, go to your health care practitioner.

CHEWING YOUR FOOD WELL

Why do we want you to chew your food well? We have teeth for a reason. Teeth are for chewing—masticating our food. We should all chew our food at least thirty-three times or until a semi-liquid forms in the mouth. This is where digestion begins, the food becomes broken down and when mixed with the saliva begins the process. As the food is moved over the tongue across the taste buds, the brain receives input about whether the food is salty, sweet, sour, bitter, meaty, savory, and so forth. Your sense of smell helps you to taste the flavor of the food. (Did you know that black licorice has no taste, only a smell?) The brain, using this information, gives the orders to begin secretion of the enzymes to aid the digestion of the food coming down the pike into the stomach.

Chewing your food is effective, not only for fat loss, but for better health. It makes sense that food that has been chewed well is easier to digest. Your stomach does not have teeth. If you drink your food, for example a protein shake, your blood sugar level is not maintained, and your body does not utilize the protein as effectively. You bypass the entire process of mastication and the normal sequence of events that occur during the process of digestion.

INDIGESTION OR ACID REFLUX

Are you taking your digestive enzymes? Are you mis-combining your food? Sometimes we may get lazy with our eating. Are you chewing each mouthful thirty-three times? Chewing is extremely important for better digestion as mastication in the mouth sets up the stomach to do its job properly. Thoroughly chewing your food will help with the digestion in your stomach, so it will likely reduce your acid reflux.

Have you waited enough time between your food groups? Did you only wait three-and-one-half hours since protein before you ate fruit? This is too early and can cause indigestion or acid reflux! WHY? Because the protein is still in your stomach and you will stop your digestion by throwing fruit on top of it! We want the stomach to empty before we consume the next food group. Food combining is very important to calm down your digestion.

LACK OF DIGESTIVE ENZYMES

Fatigue, indigestion, hiatal hernia, constipation, leg cramps, foot cramps, stomach ache, nausea, anemia, and even poor sleep can be indicators that you are lacking in digestive enzymes. If you want to lose fat, it is critical to supplement your body with digestive enzymes. Once you have been doing proper food combining for a long time, and you go into FYF4Good Phase 2, your body will adjust, and you may be able to reduce the number of digestive enzymes you take as digestion becomes stronger and more efficient. Remember that you decrease your ability to secrete digestive enzymes as you get older. Besides aging, you could have a deficiency in certain minerals.

It is important to nutrify to build muscle and make the body stronger. Hopefully you are taking a glyconutrient supplement, a whole-food multivitamin and mineral supplement, as well as the other FYF4Good recommendations, to assist your body in creating better output of your natural digestive enzymes. Do not ever forget Pillar #4: Nutrifying (see chapter two). The nutrients that are missing in the modern diet must be supplemented for building a stronger body and optimal health. We must make sure you are getting all the nutrition you need to promote rapid fat loss while supporting all cellular and bodily functions at the highest level possible.

Why does our body not produce enough digestive enzymes?

AGING: explained in the previous section!

STRESS: If you are stressed (maybe family or work issues), you are not secreting your digestive enzymes. Your body is in "Fight or Flight" mode. If you were in a forest running from a bear your body stops digestion. All the focus of the nervous system goes to the limbs. This is the same thing that happens with stress. Stress pushes blood to your limbs, increases your blood pressure, and causes dilation of your pupils so you are super alert and can see better. You might say, "Well that is silly. I am not running from a bear in the forest. I am just stressed about paying the bills." It does not matter. Stress is stress as far as your body is concerned, and digestion is on the back burner because you are running for your life as far as the body and nervous system are concerned. For this sympathetic nervous system state to occur and persist, one can understand why STRESS has been called the "silent killer." Your body goes from a relaxed, resting, functioning state of parasympathetic nervous system to fight or flight! It is very important if you can recognize what is causing your stress and then do whatever it takes to ease or alleviate it. No pill can take away the issues that cause stress. You must make other changes in your life and mindset. Try meditation, yoga, see "Pillar #7: Exercise & Sleep" in chapter two for ideas and let go of what you cannot change, do whatever it takes.

If you can only afford ONE supplement on this Lifestyle, then get the recommended digestive enzymes. If you are not breaking down your food properly, you do not have a chance of absorbing the nutrition in the food.

Your body is going to start secreting the digestive enzymes once you are food combining long enough. Eventually, you are going to be able to tell time by food combining. Four hours after your protein, you are going to get hungry. Twenty minutes after eating fruit, you are going to want to have your organic coffee, yogurt with nuts, Jackie's Chicken Salad, Jackie's Egg and Veggie Muffins, or Jackie's Three-Egg Omelet! You will know. You will feel it. The FYF4Good Lifestyle *Trains Your Brain* to understand what protein would be best to satisfy you at the time.

Your body is an amazing machine, and if we fuel it correctly everything becomes so simple. The body has memory, and eventually it will return to normal.

Pillar #4: Nutrifying (described in chapter two) is all about nutrifying with supplements. There you learned there about glyconutrient complex. They are essential for the formation of digestive enzymes. Since we do not get all of the essential glyconutrients from the foods we eat, we must supplement. Consider taking the glyconutrients for optimal results. These micronutrients are not only beneficial for the immune system, but also for cell-cell recognition. The cells must be able to recognize nutrients to bring them into the cells for optimal health and energy to burn the fat.

DIFFICULTY SLEEPING

Some people cannot stay asleep. They wake up in the middle of the night, toss and turn and cannot fall back to sleep. So what do you do if you cannot sleep? Usually you get up, shuffle around the house, and ultimately end up in the refrigerator. You eat something. Go back to bed and go right back to sleep. That is a blood sugar issue and it usually happens to people who do not eat enough protein throughout the daytime to sustain them through the night. It is very important to eat plenty of protein throughout the day. Jackie's Chicken Salad is always great! Have plenty pre-made and in serving size Tupperware ready in the refrigerator. This will assure you are never without protein.

You will not get enough protein if you skip meals or you do not have at least two to three good protein meals a day. Make sure you never let this happen. Jackie's Chicken Salad, Jackie's Three-Egg Omelet, and your goat yogurt with nuts are all great protein meals. Fruit is a nice snack to eat before you go to bed, but because of how fast it digests, if you have not eaten enough protein during the day, it will not sustain you. This is especially true if you are very hungry right before bed. On the other hand, fruit such as cherries or kiwi can sometimes be the best snack before bedtime because they contain serotonin that helps you sleep. Learning to listen to your body will help you to feed it exactly what it needs. The FYF4Good Lifestyle *Trains Your Brain* to be in control of your body.

Stress is also a factor that relates to not sleeping. Revisit "Pillar #4: Nutrifying" in chapter two for ideas on what helps reduce your stress. Try not to worry about things, especially FYF4Good. Eating according to this Lifestyle is the best possible thing you can be doing for your body. Go one meal at a time. Do not beat yourself up if you make a mistake. No one is grading you on this. It is like learning how to drive a stick shift transmission in a car. It is always touch and go until you get it down, and then you never forget and can do it practically in your sleep! Be patient and do not be hard on yourself. Go from meal to meal. Stay in present time. If you mess up, move on to the next meal and learn from the mistake.

Being in the Flush Your Fat 4Good "Buddies" Facebook Group will also help relieve stress because you will have a place to interact with trained FYF4Good Coaches and Buddies to ask questions and get helpful hints. Make sure you are connected to this group for optimal success. You will make mistakes, we all did! No worries! If you have a question about what you did, ask in the Facebook Group or contact your Buddy or Coach immediately. You can also get on our support calls.

BAD BREATH

Breath mints, gum, and lozenges will all instigate an insulin response in your body. If you are worried about your breath, get some unsweetened peppermint oil and touch it to your tongue. Also, brush your teeth after each meal to clean your mouth properly. Drink your CranFlush since that will help to clean your palate. Chew on peppermint leaves from a plant you have growing in your garden or in a pot; this is easy to do. A quick caution: make sure there are no sugars and sweeteners in your toothpaste or mouthwash. You may want to make homemade toothpaste with baking soda, Pink Himalayan Salt, peppermint oil, and water. You can add coconut oil to this mix as well, which is nice. This blend will cause your mouth to go in to an alkaline state where dental bacteria cannot proliferate. Believe it or not, we have had Buddies trigger their sugar cravings simply with the small amount of sugar or sweetener such as xylitol, contained in their toothpaste or mouthwash. This good dental hygiene will also make your dentist happy! An extra bonus!

RELEASING FLUIDS

If you feel your body is retaining fluid, try a technique called Recumbent Diuresis (elimination of fluid). A good time to do this is in the afternoon. Lay down on your couch, floor or bed. Prop your head and chest up with pillows at a forty-five-degree angle. Stretch your feet straight out in front of you, laying down outstretched. Relax in this position for at least fifteen to twenty minutes. You can read a book, watch TV, pray, answer email, make phone calls, or take a nap. Your body knows when you are resting. It slows down and relaxes. This recumbent restful position will cause the fluids to drain into your kidneys, urinary tract, and the bladder. Soon after standing up, you will need to go to the bathroom. This will help you to release excessive fluids harboring in the tissues.

HAVE I JUST HIT A PLATEAU?

Guess What? There is no such thing as a plateau in our FYF-4GOOD Lifestyle! At some point, even when you are doing everything right, your progress will appear to be slowing down. Changes do not seem to be happening as rapidly as before, but don't be fooled. This is to be expected. If your body has been rapidly losing fat and inches your brain and organs may need time to catch up. Your body may have internal repairing to do. The immune system always takes priority and might be working hard at the moment. As your body mass becomes smaller, your capillaries (extremely small blood vessels responsible for circulating blood, delivery of essential nutrients directly to tissues throughout the body, and removal of waste from those tissues) will be decreasing in number, disappearing and reabsorbed.

Over time, your heart will decrease in size from being enlarged to a more normal size relative to your new smaller body size. Hormones will be rebalancing. Your body is constantly striving to reach homeostasis, therefore, there will be healthy pauses necessary for the body to reorganize, reset, heal, repair and revise itself. There are many reasons why your body will "appear" to have plateaued. Do not get discouraged. It is expected as you slow down to make the turn into the next size of your body. Stay the course, it is all good. You are still going to be burning fat for fuel as long as you are in Nutritional Ketosis. *You Can Never Go Wrong Eating Right!*

In four months your body will have all new red blood cells. Because of the way you are eating and nutrifying your body on FYF4Good, you will be producing more healthy cells, a better copy of yourself. You are going to be stronger, healthier, and have better muscle tone. The body does not stop working. It will continue to repair itself and become healthier.

After you have lost a lot of fat, you may not see a drop in inches for two to three months, but know that you are building stronger muscles and bones. If you are still following the 8 Essential Pillars to a "T" your body is hard at work creating a healthier you! Remember, this is *A Lifestyle for a Lifetime!* Have faith in your body to build, repair and regenerate. It is possible to appear to be in a plateau for several weeks, and then experience a significant drop of inches. This should be expected. Our blood vessels must shrink, capillaries will be reabsorbed, and if the heart is enlarged it needs to shrink. Your heart is a muscle and will change size according to demand. Less body mass results in a smaller, healthier heart. Do not fight it! Your body has to readjust when it is shrinking. It may need to focus on internal repair work. You might be building lean muscle mass or increasing bone density. You really will not know what your body is doing, but you may find that you need to rest and lay down more. If that is what your body and your brain is telling you, do it!

There are some things you can do to try to help jump start and accelerate fat burning again, or to address another problem your body might be experiencing. *Read on!*

Are you walking at least five days a week, thirty minutes a day? You can walk longer, such as an hour, to continue to burn your fat. Walking longer is such a good idea if you have a sedentary job. This is a *Health Journey* as well as a fat-loss journey. If you cannot walk, do activity in your home to get your body moving. Do more activity than you have been doing. Nothing is more important than better health. Good health is one of our only real assets we can count on!

When you think you have paused in your progress or feel like you are stuck, *this* is a great time to really analyze with a fine-tooth comb, your entire day. Your journey to optimal health should not be a chore. You should feel joy and a sense of being in control. By creating a habit of eating at the proper times and having all your foods prepared ahead of time, will make this a *Habitual Ritual!* Once you get this Lifestyle down and make it your own, you will be amazed at how in charge you are of your life and your well-being. You will become your own Guru and you will be able to troubleshoot yourself to fine tune your optimal health. Surviving on this planet of ailing people, you will be the one that stands out the most for looking strong, healthy, energetic, positive and practically ageless, no matter what age you are. Your skin will glow. Your posture will be more erect. Your eyes will be more wide and bright. Your smile will be due to your internal health happiness.

Double-check yourself with these questions from time to time. Are you drinking eighty-one ounces of CranFlush? Are you food combining correctly? A common mistake is when people do not wait long enough after consuming their food groups. For example, there have been Buddies who waited three-and-one-half hours after protein, or three hours and forty-five minutes after protein instead of the full four hours before having fruit. Or, having fruit and only waiting ten or fifteen minutes before having vegetables. Make sure you wait the full four hours or longer after protein and the full twenty minutes or longer after fruit. Do not eat vegetables and then eat fruit in one hour. You must wait two hours for complete digestion of vegetables. Five minutes earlier will stop digestion because the food has not left your stomach yet and it mis-combines with the next food group. THIS IS VERY IMPORTANT!

Is every single thing you put in your mouth approved for Phase 1? Have you cheated (alcohol, birthday cake, piece of gum) in any way? Did you take a little corner piece of that coffee cake or Danish just to "taste" it?

That will stop digestion and could potentially kick you out of Nutritional Ketosis for one to four weeks. A pinch of sugar in the gas tank of your car is enough to destroy the engine! We have heard many times from Buddies that they are on a plateau but do not care because they feel so great and will never go back to how they were feeding themselves and how bad they felt. So have faith in the process and stay the course.

Double check yourself on sleep. **Are you getting enough sleep?** It should be seven to eight hours! Also, ask yourself if you are truly committed to changing your life for the better no matter what! Face yourself in the mirror and be honest with yourself. Your life and your loved ones depend on it.

I always say, that if you are not committed to changing your life for the better, up your life insurance policy for your family! —Jackie Padgette-Baird

If it has been several months, and you would like a little help to make sure you are on track, visit the private Facebook Group, or jump on a FYF4Good support call, and ask for help. ALWAYS get with your Buddy/ Coach. If you do not have a Buddy, ask for one in the Facebook Group and visit FlushYourFat4Good.com. Everyone is here to help you 24/7! What is really fun is asking your friends or family members to buddy up with you! We have some Buddies that have weekly FYF4Good pot luck meetings with Phase 1 foods. They all help each other take measurements, troubleshoot, share recipes, plus the food is GREAT! You do not have to be in the same city, state, or country. You can be and have a Buddy from anywhere.

CHAPTER ELEVEN

FYF4GOOD IS A LIFESTYLE

FOR A LIFETIME!

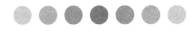

Understanding More About Eating, Digestion, and Foods

ALL SUGARS ARE NOT THE SAME
Learning About the Science of Nutrition

The most important sugars are the ones that promote GOOD HEALTH, not POOR HEALTH! Glycobiology is the study of the structure, function, and biology of saccharides (sugars) needed for life. "Glyco" derived from the Greek means sugar and, of course, "biology" is the study of life. So this relatively new science deals with the study of sugars in life. Human cells can usually synthesize the sugars found in glycans from glucose, but they are also supplied in the diet from plants.

In 2012 a group of scientists put out a call to action, asking for more research in the area of Glycobiology. Scientists are seeing the importance of sugar-containing molecules in many areas of research and the potential for them to provide scientific breakthroughs. They are even calling for this science to be taught at the high school and college levels with questions about Glycobiology being present on the SAT, MCAT, and Medical Board Exams. Many universities and other institutions have scientists doing research in this important field of study.

Currently, at least eight sugars are known to be necessary for cell-cell communication and cell-cell recognition in our bodies.

Our cells have mechanisms to make all of these sugars from those we eat, but they are not foolproof. If the body cannot make sufficient amounts of all eight sugars, breakdown of health may occur. Our immune system is extremely important in defense and protection from invader cells, cancer cells, toxins, bacteria, and parasites. Glycans on the surfaces of immune cells play important roles in defense mechanisms. For optimal health, we recommend that you take supplements of glyconutrients, mainly because we can no longer be sure that they are found in sufficient quantities in the plants that we eat. We have encountered many individuals in more than two decades who have benefited from glyconutrients supplements.

Glucose, Fructose, Sucrose, and Artificial Sweeteners

Sugars that sweeten our foods are glucose, fructose, sucrose, and "artificial sweeteners." What is the difference? Glucose, fructose, and sucrose are all "simple sugars" and are found naturally in whole foods and often added to processed foods to sweeten the flavor. All three provide the same amount of energy per gram and taste about the same. In fact, you may not be able to tell the difference by taste but make no mistake—your body can tell the difference.

Simple carbohydrates are classified as either monosaccharides or disaccharides. Monosaccharides are the simplest, most basic units of carbohydrates and are made up of only one sugar unit. Glucose and fructose are monosaccharides and are the building blocks of sucrose called a disaccharide. Thus, disaccharides are just a pair of linked sugar molecules. They are formed when two monosaccharides are joined together, and a molecule of water is removed—a dehydration reaction.

Glucose

The most important monosaccharide in this group is glucose, the body's preferred energy source. Glucose is also called blood sugar, as it circulates in the blood, and relies on enzymes to initiate metabolism. Your body processes most carbohydrates you eat into glucose, either to be used immediately for energy or to be stored in muscle cells or the liver as glycogen for later use. The hormone insulin is secreted from the pancreas primarily in response to elevated blood concentrations of glucose. Without insulin the energy source glucose will not gain entry into the cells. Diabetics are unable to adequately secrete insulin on their own and therefore are prescribed insulin by their health care practitioner to be able to get the glucose out of the blood and into the cells, reducing blood sugar to normal levels.

Fructose

Fructose is a sugar found naturally in many fruits and vegetables. It is also added to various beverages such as soda and fruit-flavored drinks most often in the form of high-fructose corn syrup. However, fructose is very different from other sugars because it has a different metabolic pathway. It is only metabolized in the liver and is not the preferred energy source for muscles or the brain. The only fructose we should be consuming on this Lifestyle is from fresh fruits and vegetables: low-glycemic (no spike in insulin) fruits and vegetables on Phase 1, all fruits and vegetables on Phase 2. Do NOT consume the refined white granular fructose sugar sold in the health food store, or the man-made high-fructose corn syrup (most corn products are GMO).

Sucrose

Sucrose is commonly known as table sugar and is obtained from sugar cane or sugar beets. Table sugar is refined and because of that, has no nutritional value whatsoever. Sucrose is the most abundant sugar in the modern diet. This is the sugar that instigates an insulin response. This is the sugar that has severe addictive properties on the brain. This is the sugar that creates a fatty liver. This is the sugar that will stop digestion. When you see sucrose or sugar on the label, put it down and step away from it. This is the sugar that can harm you.

Artificial Sweeteners

All sugars, including artificial sweeteners (artificial sugars), will trigger the brain that the body is eating sugar. It starts with the taste buds which are bundles of neuro-epithelial taste receptor cells that help the brain via the 7th, 9th, and 10th cranial nerves detect the sweet taste. The body will start to create fat. More than that, cravings will begin. Have you ever noticed people drinking diet soft drinks? Most are overfat! Diet soft drinks do not help you lose fat, in fact quite the opposite. Artificial sweeteners are not recognized by the body as real food but still trigger the brain to think it is sugar. Worse, many artificial sweeteners are dangerous to the body and have been linked to very serious health conditions. Recently, soft drink companies have started eliminating artificial sweeteners from their products. They are man-made chemicals and people are becoming educated about their dangers.

The Final Effects of So Much Sugar Consumption

The U.S. Department of Agriculture (USDA) reports that the average American consumes one 150 to 170 pounds of sugar in one year! That is one-quarter to one-half pound of sugar each day or thirty to sixty teaspoons of sugar in a twenty-four hour period! The body stores this sugar as fat. Now we can understand why obesity is epidemic and globesity is pandemic.

Sugar in fruit (fructose and glucose) is not the same as table sugar (sucrose). Table sugar (sucrose) is refined and bleached. Sucrose goes through the liver and is stored as fat on the body. Fruit has naturally occurring fructose, and when consuming low-glycemic fruits, there is no spike of insulin. A great rule of thumb is to avoid added sugars of all kinds, including artificial sweeteners (artificial sugars). This is very important; when you see on the label "No Added Sugars" that means they did not add over the 50 percent that is allowed in the product. You want "unsweetened" so that no sugars have been added at all.

On FYF4Good you will enjoy all the delicious fruits, and you will lose your cravings for sugar. We recommend that you stop eating sugar and all sweeteners in Phase 1. This means any sweetener, including Stevia, maple syrup, agave syrup, coconut sugar, mannitol, erythritol, etc., and especially the alcohol sugars: erythritol, hydrogenated starch hydrolysates, isomalt, lactitol, maltitol, Mannitol, sorbitol, and xylitol. Also known as polyols (PAH-lee-alls), sweeteners provide fewer calories than sugar and have less of an effect on blood glucose. However, many times they have a laxative effect or other gastric symptoms, especially in children. They are incompletely absorbed and metabolized. They do, however, have a positive effect because they act against tooth decay. Therefore, Phase 2 will allow gum or tooth paste with xylitol, erythritol or sorbitol if it does not negatively affect your intestines.

When you eat the FYF4Good Lifestyle, after four to five days, your sugar cravings will lessen. Soon they will disappear. When that happens, you will notice that you feel SO MUCH better, which is a blessing! On Phase 2 we teach you how to eat sweets responsibly, enjoy them immensely, but do no harm to your body. After all, living long without suffering is the goal, right?

THE DIFFERENCE BETWEEN DIABETIC KETOSIS AND NUTRITIONAL KETOSIS
These Should Never Be Confused

In a person with diabetes, dangerous and often life-threatening levels of ketones could develop. Sugar in the blood stream may soar to very high levels (hyperglycemia) and conversely, can also be dangerously low (hypo-glycemia). When sugars are too high, a diabetic might be in what is called "diabetic ketosis" (or ketoacidosis). Being in this state for long periods of time is very harmful to the body because there is too much acids (ketones) traveling through the bloodstream. If the sugars in the bloodstream are dangerously high the diabetic might lose consciousness and can actually go into what is called a "diabetic coma." If blood sugars are dangerously low, from too much insulin or not enough food, the diabetic can pass out.

Being a diabetic means your body's ability to produce and/or respond to insulin is impaired. The result is an abnormal metabolism of carbohy-drates, and high levels of glucose in the blood and urine. A diabetic must control the types of carbohydrates they put into their body and often must use insulin injections (or diabetic medicine) to regulate their body.

The Process of Nutritional Ketosis

When following Pillar #1: Nutritional Ketosis, (refer to chapter two) this should never be confused with diabetic ketosis. Nutritional Ketosis is a controlled, insulin regulated process which results in a mild release of fatty acids and ketone production in response to a reduction in carbohydrate intake. Insulin is still secreted but at very low sustained levels because the foods we consume do not cause an insulin response or spike.

A person with diabetic ketosis (ketoacidosis) is starving to death and is a medical concern. Ketoacidosis is driven by a lack of insulin in the body. Without insulin the muscle, fat and liver cells become less permeable to receiving glucose and the body cannot efficiently turn glucose into glycogen. Glycogen is a multi-branched polysaccharide of glucose that serves as a form of energy storage in the liver and muscles. Glycogen represents the main storage form of glucose in the body.

Think of it this way: When the diabetic's body runs out of glycogen, it triggers the production of ketones from fats and amino acids to prevent starvation. Because insulin is not produced normally in the diabetic's body, glucose cannot gain entrance into the cells and it cannot be converted effectively to glycogen. Therefore, there is excess glucose in the bloodstream. The production of ketones does not stop, flooding the blood stream with ketones until the diabetic becomes ill from ketoacidosis (too much acid in the bloodstream). The breath of a diabetic, in this situation, can actually smell similar to acetone or sweet like alcohol, due to ketones. This can be an indicator that the diabetic is getting into trouble. When this happens, the diabetic starves to death because they cannot get glycogen to their brain. Remember, insulin is needed to turn glucose into glycogen. The diabetic does make insulin, but in type 2 there is resistance to it. In type 1 the beta cells in the pancreas may be wiped out and then there would be no insulin. Ninety percent of diabetics are type 2.

People who secrete small amounts of insulin will not go into a starvation ketoacidosis. The body will go into Keto Adaptation or Nutritional Ketosis. This is where the body will start breaking down the fat to produce glycogen. The stored fat is burned for fuel! The unique Lifestyle of Phase 1 and Phase 2 of FYF4Good is all inclusive with a broad spectrum of foods that many diets that focus on fat burning do not allow. FYF4Good is focused on digestion, absorption and elimination, with low-glycemic fruits and vegetables. Add food combining and it not only becomes fun but greatly improves your health.

Is Nutritional Ketosis safe for a diabetic?

Diabetics do very well on the FYF4Good Lifestyle! Of course, it is recommended that diabetics review FYF4Good and consult with their health care practitioner before starting. As your health starts to improve, your blood sugars values may start to change, making it necessary for your health care practitioner to adjust your medications as the fat is rapidly shed. This is a GOOD THING!

THE DIGESTIVE SYSTEM

The Digestive System (the process of digestion) begins in the mouth and ends at your bottom or, more specifically, the anatomical word is the *anus*.

Do you remember your mother saying, "do not eat so fast" or "chew your food before you swallow it"? Her advice was spot-on. Keep in mind that your stomach does not have teeth. Chewing food before swallowing helps to breakdown the food into a thick liquid, called bolus, necessary for proper digestive processing. It also signals the body to start producing the right digestive enzymes to digest the type of food we are eating.

Most people, even as adults, do not chew long enough. When you have chewed your food properly, there should be very little left to swallow. It should almost feel like it has dissolved in your mouth. FYF4Good recommends you chew each bite of food at least thirty-three times! Yes, thirty-three times! Most people chew three to seven times and then swallow whole pieces of food. This will not encourage optimal digestion, absorption, and elimination!

What is even more fascinating is that every twenty-four hours we produce approximately thirty ounces of saliva from the tiny glands in our mouth and jaw. As we chew our food, saliva starts the breakdown of the food, as well as lubricates the food to help it move through the digestive tract. Salivating just at the sight, smell or thought of certain foods is a normal physiological response because the nerves that control the saliva production are part of a reflex system.

Remember the Pavlov dog experiments? Pavlov proved that sight and smell, and in the case of humans, the very thought of food, will trigger salivation. These nerves will fire without you even consciously knowing it. The movement of your jaw muscle can activate the reflex. A signal is sent to the primary salivary center in the medulla oblongata, located in the brainstem. This signal gets the party started by releasing neurotransmitters such as acetylcholine and norepinephrine. These chemicals initiate nerve signals telling the glands to produce saliva. Digestion starts in the mouth but for some people, we could argue it starts in the brain. This is all automatic. We do not have to think about it.

The food leaves our **mouth** to go through the **throat (pharynx)** into the **esophagus,** a muscular contracting tube that delivers the food to the **stomach**. At the very end of the esophagus is a valve called the lower esophageal sphincter. It keeps the food from traveling back out of the stomach into the esophagus. Our body has a "wave" called peristalsis, starting with the esophagus, which propels the food all the way through the long digestive tract. Peristalsis causes the hunger pangs or stomach "growling" we sometimes hear.

Once the food is in the stomach, the strong muscular walls of the stomach contract to mix the food with heat acid and powerful digestive enzymes. When the food is ready to leave the stomach, it has the consistency of a liquid or paste and is called chyme.

Continuing down the digestive tract, the next section after the stomach is the small intestine. The small intestine, like the esophagus, contracts to move the food along. This section is about twenty feet long and has three parts: the **duodenum**, the **jejunum** and the **ileum**. In the duodenum, the food continues to be broken down with digestive enzymes released from the pancreas and bile from the liver. Bile cleans waste products from the blood and aids in breaking down fat. The jejunum and the ileum are mainly responsible for absorbing the nutrients into the bloodstream.

There are three organs in our body that help the stomach and small intestine break down and digest the food we eat. The **pancreas** secretes digestive enzymes into the small intestine to break down protein, fat and carbohydrates. Two functions of the **liver** that help our digestive system are to make the bile, and to clean the blood coming from the small intestine (containing the newly absorbed nutrients). Sitting below the liver is the **gallbladder,** the storage tank for the bile. Bile is needed to digest fats. The gallbladder delivers the bile into the small intestine through the bile duct.

Once the food travels thru the small intestine, anything remaining that has not been absorbed goes into the **large intestine** (also known as the colon). At this point, what was once known as food is now referred to as "stool," "feces," or "waste" (food product and bacteria). The colon really has nothing to do with absorption of nutrients from foods. The **colon** is about five feet long and three inches in diameter and contracts to move the stool, which is in a liquid state. As it is moving, the colon removes and absorbs the liquid (water) as well as ions and nutrients from gut bacteria and stores the solid remains in the sigmoid colon. Two or three times a day this empties into the rectum where the process of elimination begins.

The job of the **rectum** is to receive the stool from the colon, signal your body that it is ready to be evacuated and hold it until the evacuation happens. The **anus** is the anatomical end of the digestive tract. It provides the final control to keep the body from evacuating the stool until ready. It takes approximately twenty-four to seventy-two hours for food to get from the mouth to the rectum in a normal healthy adult. Doesn't it make sense to eat only healthy, clean foods that travel from the mouth to the anus to protect the entire system?

What happens in the digestive tract when you mis-combine your food?

Here is a typical scenario of what happens physiologically with digestion when you do NOT combine your foods properly as FYF4Good recommends. As you chew, there are certain acid enzymes that will be produced immediately upon detection of protein. When you eat a bite of Jackie's Chicken Salad, these powerful acid enzymes will be secreted. Now imagine that you wanted a piece of bread with your meal, because you just had to have it (this is a mis-combining of your foods). As you chew the bread, your brain detects starch while it is in your mouth. It immediately stops digestion of the protein and orders the pancreas to secrete the appropriate alkaline enzymes to digest that bread. Peristalsis is also slowed or halted. NOT GOOD!

Chemistry 101: When you put an alkaline and an acid in a beaker, they neutralize each other and become ineffective. The same thing happens in the stomach. The Jackie's Chicken Salad and the bread (starch) are sitting there while the stomach is churning, churning, churning. Since the acid and alkaline have neutralized each other, there are no enzymes present that can digest and assimilate the foods.

The stomach, in its strenuous efforts, can allow acid to creep up through the esophageal sphincter or valve. Presto! Gastric reflux and heartburn are born. Some familiar chronic conditions for this have been named GERD (gastric esophageal reflux disorder) or Hiatal Hernia Syndrome. They are not fun and can be very painful, sometimes feeling like a heart attack. This feeling can take your breath away as well as burn in the stomach and up in the esophagus, sometimes including uncomfortable belching and gas.

Overtime, the gastric reflux can eventually cause destruction of the esophagus due to regurgitation of stomach acids back up into the esophagus, and "burn" or damage the distal esophagus where it empties into the stomach. Have you noticed all of the TV commercials promoting antacids? People take antacids to try to stop the burning and belching. This is simply a Band-Aid, taking care of symptoms, but does not solve the problem.

What they commonly need are more digestive enzymes and food combining! The stomach in this case is ineffective due to low levels of digestive enzyme production because we lose the ability to make adequate digestive enzymes as we get older. While the stomach continues to try to break down the food contents, reflux and regurgitation occurs up through the hiatal sphincter as the stomach works very hard to breakdown the food. Digestive enzyme supplementation aids the stomach to effectively breakdown the food preventing the regurgitation episodes.

At some point, the reflux can get so bad that surgery is recommended by doctors. By combining your foods properly (refer to "Pillar #2: Food Combining" in chapter two) and supplementing with the important appropriate nutrients (refer to "Pillar #4: Nutrifying" in chapter two), this scenario improves tremendously and, in most cases, stops. That extra burden of the digestive tract is removed, and the neutralization of acid and alkaline enzymes does not occur. FYF4Good takes the burden off the digestive tract, creating optimal digestion. You will not really understand how bad you have felt until your digestion is finally working optimally, and you feel great!

HOW TO FIND A NEW TASTE YOU LOVE IN TEN DAYS
Reprogramming Your Taste Buds
If you are dealing with a small child, who does not understand or care about nutritional benefits, and will not eat their vegetables, understanding

WHY they do not like something may be helpful. Is it the taste, the temperature or the texture? Presenting the food in another manner, (mixed with other tasty foods, blended in a sauce, etc.) may result in success in getting the nutrients into your child's body.

But as adults, do we really need to blend our food together to disguise goat yogurt, kale or coffee? The answer is NO. It takes only ten days to reprogram your taste buds and it is very easy to do. Take for example goat yogurt. On occasion, one of our Buddies would swear they cannot consume goat yogurt because they have never had it before and it tastes different. They say they do not like it. Some even say that it makes them gag.

Most of us eat the same few foods all the time, so when we try a new food, we must acquire a taste for it. Did you know you can reprogram your taste buds to like, and possibly love, goat yogurt or any other food, in ten days?

On the back of your tongue you have taste buds for bitter tastes. On the sides of your tongue you taste sour flavors. At the tip of your tongue you taste sweet and salty flavors. But located in the very center of your tongue, are very few taste buds. When learning to like a new food, avoid the bitter, sour, sweet, and salt taste buds and start with the center of your tongue.

Let us say you believe you do not like goat yogurt. Take a very tiny amount, maybe one-eighth to one-quarter of a teaspoon of goat yogurt. Place this on the center of your tongue and hold it there as the saliva will start to surround your yogurt before swallowing. Try starting with just fifteen seconds the first day. Let it dissolve and then swallow it. This will trigger the brain to understand that it is good for your body. Each day (or try twice a day if you want to move faster), increase the time and the amount of goat yogurt held in your mouth before swallowing.

If this is not working for you, dip one of your soaked nuts, such as a walnut, into the goat yogurt. Get just a little goat yogurt on it and place it on the center of your tongue. Just hold it there for ten seconds and then chew thoroughly and swallow it. Repeat until it becomes easy. Then increase the amount of goat yogurt to one-half or even three-quarters of a teaspoon and do the same thing. You will be shocked at how quickly the brain will acquire the taste for it. Some people eat the goat yogurt with nuts with a little pure vanilla (no sugars or sweeteners added), cinnamon or even cayenne pepper. But first, let your brain enjoy plain!

Most Buddies who were not sure they liked goat yogurt and said it made them gag, were shocked and pleased to acquire the taste for it. They now enjoy goat yogurt mixed with soaked walnuts or pecans. Some also enjoy goat yogurt with diced cucumbers, red onions and a little dill weed. They cannot wait for this part of their daily routine and find it a surprisingly delicious, fresh tasting treat. The benefits of goat yogurt for your body make it well worth it. You, too, can look forward to this!

READING THE LABEL: WHOLE-FOOD VERSUS SYNTHETIC SUPPLEMENTATION

Most supplements on the market are synthetic! Over 90 percent!

As we have explained, synthetic vitamins are made from coal tar, petroleum, petroleum by-products, ground-up rocks, iron shavings and/or chemicals. Minerals are mined from the ground and processed into fine powders. No matter how fine the powder, they are not in a form that can be processed by the human body. Synthetic vitamins are not made from natural food.

With FYF4Good, we are always looking for the *best* supplements to feed our bodies. Check FlushYourFat4Good.com for current recommendations on supplements and sources for those products.

How do you identify whole-food versus synthetic supplements?

When reading a supplement label, whole-food vitamins and minerals will often include parentheses next to the nutrient indicating the food source for the vitamin or mineral. Synthetic nutrition may say USP (US Pharmaceutical) Grade as well as there will be certain key words that will give it away.

For example, vitamin C occurs naturally in citrus fruits, rose hips, spinach, broccoli, tomatoes, and acerola cherries. If you see any of these listed on the label, the vitamin C is coming from a food source. Vitamin C complex contains rutin, flavonoids, catechin, polyphenols, several enzymes, and more. Synthetically, it comes to us as ascorbic acid. If you see ascorbic acid on the label, that is synthetic, and not the entire vitamin complex.

Whole-Food Supplementation is BETTER

Nutritional supplements from whole-food have a higher bioavailability. This means that when they make it to your small intestine, they will absorb into your blood stream more effectively and have greater benefit to the body. Therefore, when you consume nutrition from a food source, you do not need as much quantity of the nutrition as you do when you ingest it in the form of synthetic supplement.

Whole-food supplements also come in the complete food matrix; thus your body will be able to recognize it and use it properly.

So just because a synthetic nutritional supplement has more quantity, do not be fooled into thinking you will get more into your body, and therefore it must be better.

Warnings About Synthetic Nutritional Supplements

A warning of caution when consuming synthetic substitutes: Some have been shown to have harmful effects on the body. The *New England Journal of Medicine* in 1995 and 1996 reported the results of studies on synthetic nutrition and its harmful effects. These studies showed that certain synthetic vitamins:

Increased lung cancer rates by 46 percent

Increased cardiovascular disease by 26 percent

Increased mortality rates in forty-seven (47) clinical trials

Increased birth defects by 400 percent!

A European study showed that the risk of heart attack is doubled if too much calcium is consumed.

Do Not Be Fooled!

You may see the word "natural" on some synthetic supplement labels. This is a marketing claim. Arsenic is natural! Since the FDA and USDA do not have a definition of the word "natural," up to 90 percent of that product can legally be synthetic. Also, coal tar, petroleum, and ground-up rocks are "natural," since they occur in nature, but they are not food.

Many supplements that are marketed as "natural" contain synthetic parts to standardize the amounts of nutrition in the product. Synthetic is still synthetic. Again, do not be fooled!

How to Read the Label

The following chart will help you to identify whole-food versus synthetic sources. This chart is not a complete list but should contain enough information to help you identify most synthetic supplements.

Vitamins ending in any of these words are synthetic: Palmitate, Acetate, Mononitrate, Hydrochloride, or Succinate.

Minerals not from food sources usually have words ending in -ide and -ate. Examples: ascorbate, carbonate, citrate, aspartate, gluconate, sulfate, chloride, iodide, disulfide, and oxide.

Vitamin	Natural	Synthetic
A	Cod Liver Fish Oils, Carrots	Acetate, Palmitate
B	Yeast	Thiamine, Mononitrate, Thiamine Hydrochloride, Riboflavin, Pyridoxine Hydrochloride
C	Citrus, Rose Hips, Spinach, Broccoli, Tomatoes, Acerola Berries	Ascorbic Acid
D	Cod Liver Fish Oils	Irradiated Ergosteral, Calciferol
E	D-alpha Tocopherol, Wheat Germ Oil	Dl-alpha Tocopherol
K	Green leafy vegetables, oils	Menadione, Phytonadione
Biotin	Liver	D-biotin
Choline	Soy Beans	Choline Chloride, Choline Bitartrate
Folic Acid	Yeast, Liver	Pteroylglutamic Acid
Niacin	Yeast	Niacin
Pantothenic Acid	Rice Bran, Yeast	Calcium D-Pantothenate
Beta-carotene	Carrot, Sweet Potato	Petrochemicals, (benzene from acetylene gas)

HOW MUCH PROTEIN ARE WE SHOOTING FOR IN A DAY?

On FYF4Good we do not measure. We recommend Jackie's Three-Egg Omelet in the morning or Jackie's Egg and Veggie Muffins or goat yogurt with nuts. Some people eat Jackie's Chicken Salad or other protein such as salmon for their first protein meal. FYF4Good, when followed to a "T," Re-*Trains Your Brain* to signal your body what it needs, including what and how much to eat. Some days you will want a four-egg omelet or a second serving of goat yogurt with nuts. Some days you will want a two-egg omelet. All of this is Okay. *Do Not Overeat! Do Not Under-Eat!* For many of us our brains have been on vacation, so they need to be retrained. We want to be able to know when we are full, when we have had enough, or when we need to eat more just by listening to our brain. You will know and become so in tune with your body that for the first time in your life, you may push yourself away from the table after only eating half of the food on the plate, getting the message from somewhere inside that you have had enough. This is when you know YOU ARE IN CONTROL…THE BRAIN HAS TAKEN OVER, as it should. It is truly a wondrous moment to learn your food no longer has control over you!

If you are experiencing sugar cravings, or you cannot sleep through the night, it could mean that you are not eating enough protein. Did you skip a meal or are you eating very small portions? You will already know in your heart if you are not eating enough. It will become obvious to you. So listen and follow! Remember, FYF4Good is not about portion control!

With Jackie's Chicken Salad, you are supposed to eat enough until you are full and satisfied. Jackie herself has been known to eat several bowls in one sitting. She NEEDED it! If you need more, eat more. As you lose fat and get smaller, you will probably need less. And you will have days when your body will be working on something and you will want to eat a lot more. Other days, you may want to eat quite a bit less. This is absolutely normal. Babies and young children do this all the time. When they are growing they eat more, and when they are not, they do not want to eat as much. The brain is in control and they are functioning with their innate intelligence. The one rule we have is to eat at least a little to keep the blood sugar up, preventing it from dramatically dropping. This is like throwing kindling on the campfire. By eating and not missing meals, you will keep the metabolism optimally burning the fat for fuel.

Some of you are still going to want a number of grams of protein needed each day. We do not measure it. Everyone is different. However, for the recommended daily allowance (RDA), you can multiply your weight in pounds by 0.36 and that will give you just a ball park figure of the amount of grams of protein for an average day. More importantly, on FYF4Good you will start to know and feel that you should have more. Listen to your brain. On Phase 1 eat protein throughout the day. In other words, instead of just a green salad, we want you to add protein to it with each meal. That is why Jackie's Chicken/Egg/Turkey/Tuna (tofu for vegetarians) Salad is great as you get all you need in that one bowl of salad. *Note*: Vegetarians eating Jackie's Tofu Salad can include nuts and seeds, as these are both plant proteins. Do not blend plant proteins with animal proteins.

For people that are overfat and have been eating starches and sugar, the brain was completely on "vacation." The brain must take charge again, like it was when we were babies. When breast-feeding, babies stop eating when they are full because their satiety center is signaled from the brain. There is absolutely no way to measure how much milk that baby ate. When bottle feeding, parents are trying to estimate how many ounces the baby should be eating at each meal as compared to last meal or yesterday, and then proceed to try to "stuff" the baby if they did not eat very much at that sitting. In babies, their innate brain function triggers the satiety (a feeling of being full). Over-stuffing the baby becomes the beginning of the overeating paradigm.

With FYF4Good we give the job of digestion, absorption, and elimination back to the brain. The brain controls and coordinates ALL functions in the human body. So many of us were taught to overeat for comfort and to clean our plates or we will be punished because all the poor people are starving when we are so lucky, and so on. As we have said, these are paradigms that have been passed on from generation to generation. Much of this came from people who lived through the Depression or other hard times when food was scarce. But with the proper food choices, we stop the chaos of the insulin hormone rollercoaster, and we put the brain back in charge. You will know because you will be energized, and you will have a true sense of well-being.

SELECTING FRUITS and VEGETABLES

On Phase 1, select fruits and vegetables with a **glycemic index (GI) of sixty (60 GI) or lower**. Following is a quick reference list of some of the most common fruits and vegetables enjoyed on FYF4Good. Others are good too. Use your internet search engine to check the glycemic index on fruits and vegetables before you buy. When you soften certain vegetables (e.g. carrots or tomatoes), by cooking them, they turn to high-glycemic, so be careful. And a great tip is *The Harder to Chew, The More You Lose!*

Low-glycemic index means the sugar will be absorbed slower and will not instigate an insulin response or spiking of insulin from your pancreas. The higher the GI score, the quicker the sugar is absorbed into the blood, causing a blood sugar spike. For reduced sugar cravings, and for maximum fat burning, pick foods with a lower GI score.

Glycemic load (GL) of food is a number that estimates how much the food will raise a person's blood glucose level after eating it. GL is based on the **glycemic index** (**GI**) and is calculated by multiplying the grams of available carbohydrate in the food, times the food's **GI** and then dividing by one hundred. We do not worry about this as the brain tells you when enough is enough; especially with low-glycemic eating and food combining. Listen to your body. You will be amazed at what you hear. It is also amazing that after about seventy-two hours to about two weeks of FYF4Good, most of you will have eliminated your craving for sugar and you will be running to the kitchen for your fruit!

On Phase 1, do not have fruit juices or vegetable juices, except for unsweetened, not from concentrate 100 percent cranberry juice that is recommended and the CranFlush or ginger that has been freshly juiced for CranGingerFlush.

Fruit	Glycemic Index		Vegetable	Glycemic Index
Apple	39		Artichoke	15
Apricot	57		Asparagus	14
Blackberries	32		Bell Peppers	10
Blueberries	40		Broccoli	10
Cherries	22		Brussels Sprouts	16
Grapes	46		Carrot	47
Kiwi	52		Cauliflower	15
Mango	56		Celery	15
Papaya	55		Cucumber	15
Peach	42		Green Beans	14
Pear	58		Mushroom	10
Plum	38		Onion	10
Raspberries	32		Tomato	15
Strawberry	40		Zucchini	11

No bananas, avocados, melons, or dried fruits on Phase 1. Even though their GI scores are low, they contain very little water and will slow down digestion. We are interested in rapid fat loss. This is *FLUSH Your Fat, not SLUSH Your Fat!* Fruits with more fluid move easier in the gut and help maximize digestion. The goal of Phase 1 is to get the digestion working properly again and to get the fat off as quickly as possible and 4Good!

Most people have a very sluggish digestive tract and have had this, knowingly or unknowingly, for a very long time. On Phase 2, if you are going to eat a banana, eat it last, following all your other fruits, and then wait thirty minutes for digestion (instead of twenty minutes) before you change food groups. Remember, no bananas on Phase 1. They are saved for Phase 2. This goes for avocados as well. Just like the banana, it is a wonderful healthy food, but it has no fluids and therefore slows down digestion.

Non-Starchy Vegetables

ONLY eat non-starchy vegetables. Following is a partial list. Use your internet search engine to find others (type in search window "Is/Are

_____ a starch?"). Keep in mind that certain non-starchy, low-glycemic vegetables, such as carrots and tomatoes become high-glycemic when they are cooked. Remember, *The Harder to Chew, the More You Lose!*

Alfalfa Sprouts	Carrots	Jicama	Peppers	*Types of Squash:*
Arugula	Cauliflower	Kale	Radishes	*Cushaw*
Artichoke	Celery	Leeks	Romaine	*Summer*
Asparagus	Cucumber	Mushrooms	Sprouts	*Crookneck*
Broccoli	Eggplant	Okra	Swiss Chard	*Spaghetti*
Brussels Sprouts	Green Onions	Onions	Tomato	*Zucchini*

Cruciferous Vegetables Need Special Care

Cruciferous vegetables have cancer-fighting nutrients as well as other tremendous health benefits, but some of these vegetables can be hard to digest when eaten raw. Slightly steaming or grilling broccoli, Brussels sprouts, and cauliflower, for example, helps to break down the fibers and promote ease of digestion.

One exception with broccoli occurs when it is added to Jackie's Chicken Salad. We are only using the florets and not the stems, chopping them up into very small pieces for the salad and letting them marinate in the lemon and mayonnaise. Since the florets are chopped finely, this will allow for easier digestion. Some people also feel they want to slightly steam their kale. However, you are not eating mounds of it in Jackie's Chicken Salad so doing this may be overkill.

Cruciferous vegetables include arugula, Brussels sprouts, cauliflower, broccoli, cabbage, kale, rutabaga, and more. Use your internet search engine to check for others.

Most people have not been eating enough fruits and vegetables. You will do yourself a favor if you learn to eat plenty of both. Just keep them low-glycemic and non-starchy, as well as organic when possible. You will begin to notice how much better you feel just by eating these healthy foods on a daily basis. You will come to "know" they are really nourishing your body.

So let us say it one more time! FYF4Good is not a diet. It is *A Lifestyle for a Lifetime.* By following the FYF4Good Lifestyle, you will have all the knowledge and power to be lean and healthy for life and to never struggle again.

AFTERWORD

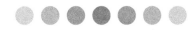

Please visit FlushYourFat4Good.com for more information about following the FYF4Good *Lifestyle*, including available online courses and services, the schedule for live support calls and events, great recipes, FAQs, our Flush Your Fat 4Good Workbook, and helpful charts (Low-Glycemic Fruits and Vegetables, A-Day-at-a-Glance for Phase 1, Diminishing Measurements). You can also find recommendations on where to find high quality supplements and so much more!

ABOUT THE AUTHORS

JACKIE PADGETTE-BAIRD

Frogs were ALWAYS around our house when I was growing up. You see, my father was the first bio-analyst and pathologist in the State of California. He discovered the use of African Frogs for pregnancy tests in the 1950s. To sit at the breakfast table with this man was a trip. "Mastication," "digestion," "clean out your liver with hot water, lemon and a pinch of salt," and "chew your foods, since your stomach doesn't have teeth," were the topic of conversation daily. No kid is really interested in that stuff, but that didn't matter. We heard about our bodies all the time! It was not until later in my life that I would come to realize how truly blessed I was to have my father's influence instigate a healthier survival.

Time with my father was way too short! He spent time living with the Masai and Ubangi tribes in Africa. He not only helped them decrease the rate of childbirth deaths by teaching them about how and why the birth environment should be sanitary, but he also hunted with them for food. On one such trip, we believe my father was bitten by a tsetse fly. He developed cerebral malaria and passed away when I was only eight and a half years old. In that very short time I had with him, the seeds of my interests in biochemistry and real nutrition were planted in my mind.

My mother was a gourmet cook and was interested in nutrition. My siblings and I would beg for sugary, store-bought cookies and cakes, but she insisted on making healthy ones for us. She would turn Jack LaLanne on the television and preach how we all needed to get up and exercise.

Something must have sunk in, because in high school I became a gymnast and studied dance.

My obsession with music started at twelve when I began playing the guitar. By fourteen I was teaching others how to play. At fifteen, my fraternal twin sister, Spice, and I began performing together. We made a big splash locally and loved it. Spice called me a few years after high school about a musical group needing musicians and singers. I immediately said "NO!" but she talked me into auditioning. Actually, she threatened me, but that's another story. That was the beginning of my wild and crazy journey of adventure, love, and success in the music industry as Sugar 'n Spice. This is where I met my soul mate and first husband, Dick Padgette, the bass player and leader of our group.

Being on the road as a musician, singer, and songwriter for many years was grueling on my body. There was little time to sleep, and less time for eating healthy. I was often sick but still needed to sing, dance and play guitar as we performed all over the country. All doctors could do for me during this time was give me drugs - for the pain, to go to sleep, to feel better - you name it, they were giving it to me. The more pills I swallowed, the more problems I was having. A loud voice in my head started screaming at me that I had better learn as much as I could about survival, or I wouldn't make it. This is when I realized doctors practice medicine, but they don't practice health.

Don't get me wrong! We need doctors. If I break my leg, don't take me to the health food store first! Take me to the emergency room and a doctor who knows how to set bones. But I knew if I had to rely on doctors fidgeting with different drugs to offset my exhaustion and poor eating habits, I'd be in serious trouble. So I went to the library, the health food store, medical journals, anywhere I could, and started my own quest for optimal health and well-being. I found so many incredible science/nutrition books, including one that was all about food combining! This changed my life forever! I became entrenched with the knowledge of how to survive on our ailing planet. It was during this time that it hit me: optimal health and well-being had been part of my entire life. It started with my father around that kitchen table.

In the mid-'80s I was cutting albums, singing back-up for amazing artists and making a name for myself in the music industry. Man, I was going for it. As a girl guitarist, singer, and songwriter, I was living the life! And then I got pregnant with my first son. At four months along I was in a serious car crash. Not one chiropractor would touch me because it was believed that "adjusting" a pregnant woman would put her into labor. But I was in pain, so I was persistent in looking for help. Finally, I was introduced to Dr. Victoria Arcadi, who specialized in pregnancy and newborns. She performed miracles for me to feel better and get right back into the swing of things.

In the early '90s, six months after giving birth to my second son, my manager wanted me to go to Germany where my music was really appreciated. The kicker was that I had to go there by myself and leave my family in the states. This idea tortured me until I realized I could lay down and die knowing I gave up my career, but I could never forgive myself knowing I gave up my family. So I left the music industry to follow my second love in life, NUTRITION.

I started working as a Chiropractic Assistant for Dr. Vicky and loved helping with her research, studying and understanding supplements, and working with patients. In 1994, pregnant with my third child (a daughter this time!), California was hit with one of the biggest earthquakes of all time, the Northridge Earthquake. Reseda/Northridge, where I lived, was on the epicenter. As the earthquake struck, I fell over a bookcase trying to protect my two boys. This trauma blew a hole in my daughter's heart, and I had to remain bedridden until she was born. With the help of Dr. Vicky and my midwife, during the last month of pregnancy her heart grew back together, and she was born weighing ten pounds, healthy and beautiful.

Despite the joy of the new addition to our family, life was a real struggle due to the earthquake's damage. This is when Dr. Vicky and I decided to form a partnership to focus full-time on a nutrition business. The business took off, and we were helping so many people get healthy. We were getting our feet back under us from all the expenses and stress caused by the earthquake. I could see the light at the end of the tunnel…and then it all exploded. I lost my husband of thirty years to lung and brain cancer. He was my soul mate. I did not have much time to mourn as I had three kids to care for and needed to be strong for them, but I felt like I lost my right arm.

As God would have it, though, I met and married my second husband and felt so blessed to have had a second time around with such a wonderful man, Tom Baird. He adopted my kids and loved them as his own and taught them all how to surf. But time was too short. After only eleven years of marriage, Tom passed away and I became a two-time widow with three kids. It was all I could do to just concentrate on the nutrition business with Dr. Vicky to support my family and move forward in life. So I did.

If Tom's death was not hard enough to bear, another tragedy took almost everything out of me. My beautiful little girl was bullied at school in the sixth grade and then started using drugs. The time, energy, guilt, and fear of what could happen led me down a road of constant sleeplessness and erratic eating. I will never give up on my kids. I studied and researched all I could find. We tried programs and counseling, but nothing was working. I was determined to make her well and eventually found a clinic outside of the US that allowed me to finally feel safe, hopeful, and at peace. I was able to get my daughter the help she needed, and after checking her in I was able to sleep straight through the night for the first time in a very, very long time. Amazing what a good night's sleep can do for you.

When I awoke, I was so grateful and happy. I went to my bathroom mirror, took one look at myself and said, "Oh, hell no! How did all that weight get on me? Oh My God! This fat has got to go, like yesterday!" I knew how fifty-plus pounds got on me: stress, erratic eating, and very little sleep, but it was a shock to see it! It was now my turn to care for myself and I needed to get the fat off fast.

Being educated in science/nutrition, supplementing, and eating in a healthy way was in my favor, but as we all know, dieting is horrible because of the feelings of deprivation and fatigue and is something none of us do very consistently. The thought of dieting, getting some of it off, and then gaining it back as everyone always does, only to start all over again, was horrifying to me!

I walked around the house a couple of times feeling really disturbed by this and started talking to myself: "What am I going to do now?" I went into the kitchen and stood in front of my pantry, bewildered. "How long is this going to take? How could I not have seen this happen to me? Can I easily get it off at my age?" I was terribly upset, as I know just twenty pounds of fat on your body is linked to over twenty health conditions. I needed to become healthy and strong for my kids. They had already lost two dads and I needed to be there for them.

I was seriously deep in thought when I heard His voice: "Jackie, you know what to do." I kid you not, when I say I heard HIS voice. I even turned around to look and see who was in the kitchen with me. The good Lord was whispering in my right ear. "You have all the knowledge and now it is time to put it into action." Within twenty minutes, FYF4Good was completely downloaded into my brain and I proceeded to apply it to myself like a robot. I knew exactly what to do, when to do it, and what to take to make all the fat melt off me in order to give me the strength and the energy to enjoy the process.

After a few weeks of my privately applying all the knowledge given to me by Divine Intervention, I was shocking my friends. They could not believe how fast the fat was just melting off me. I felt amazingly strong, energized, and happy. A friend, Cathy Castelazo, insisted I put it down on paper for her clients in her health business. She started getting amazing results with her clients.

Dr. Vicky, my business partner and dear friend, realized we needed to study the plan, so we developed two trial groups of approximately twenty people each for twelve weeks. The results were breathtaking. Everyone's lives were rapidly changing, just as promised to me that day in my kitchen. *Health by Design, Not by Default!*

Making this *A Lifestyle for a Lifetime* is honoring the body that God has given us. To appreciate our lives and the quality of our health is the most important thing we have. Flush Your Fat 4Good: *Be Lean and Healthy for Life* is our motto and our creed. Changing people's relationship with their food and learning how to live a long, vibrant, and healthy life is what FYF4Good is all about.

DR. VICTORIA C. ARCADI

I do not think there can be any argument about the state of the world in regard to obesity. It is everywhere, and it is pandemic. So much so, that there is a term for it now—GLOBESITY, or "global obesity."

I was an innocent child affected by the "trickle-down" effect from family obesity. It was like watching a very slow, tortuous, and miserable death. As a child, I had to endure my mother's obesity. I was a casualty. Watching the progression of this curse was truly horrible for all the loved ones around her.

My mother was a prodigy, gifted violinist and full of life. Because she was gregarious and outgoing with personality-plus she was the perfect person to invite to your party to help to make it fun and successful. She was also smart, worldly, and incredibly intelligent with regard to almost every subject.

But as a result of the bondage in her body after the birth of her children, she had uncontrollable weight gain along with depression, feeling uncomfortable and unwell, self-suppression, embarrassment, self-conscious loathing of her looks, and she became miserable. She put on a good show because she loved to socialize, as she sadly developed marked physical limitations, low self-esteem, and feelings of doom and gloom, which eventually made her unable to do many of the things mothers and daughters do together. I missed many of the joys with my mother that most people take for granted, such as spending the day shopping and then going out to lunch, or attending my college tennis matches and tournaments, walking our dogs around a beautiful golf course, going to the beach and walking in the waves, getting on a plane and taking a holiday, or even spontaneously taking off and going to the movie theater.

My mother tried all the different fads, pills, Optifast, starvation diets, grapefruit diet, watermelon diet, shots, Scarsdale Diet, hormones—you name it—throughout her life and mine. All her efforts backfired because with each attempt to lose the weight, while it often appeared that it was working, the diet ultimately resulted in her gaining all of the weight back—plus a lot more. Not to mention that the starvation diets are known to be dangerous for the health of the heart as the body cannibalizes itself from its muscles, including the heart, to take care of the needs of the body.

The sequelae associated with obesity (twenty pounds or more overfat) in various degrees is slowed metabolism, consistent weight gain, arthritic changes in the knees, hips, and spine, high blood pressure, edema, a pre-diabetic condition or full-blown diabetes, inflammation, the need for a wheelchair and then, ultimately, congestive heart failure. I watched my mom travel this path and spiral downward over the course of my lifetime until her death when I was fifty.

As a thirty-plus year family practitioner of chiropractic, I helped to manage my mother's last ten months in hospice with end-stage congestive heart failure. It was a blessing that after being bed-bound for ten years due to severe arthritic changes in her hips, knees and feet caused by morbid obesity, in her last ten months she lost all the excess weight. She went on a special diet limiting starches, sugars, and cow dairy. While in hospice and bedridden, I handed her caregiver a manual that showed what and when she was to eat along with a schedule of when and how to take the nutritional supplements to nutrify her body.

As the fat was pouring off her body, the hospice team was flabbergasted because she continued to be titrated down on her medications. Water retention, which is very severe with congestive heart failure, improved until she was titrated completely off her diuretic medication. Her blood pressure returned to normal, and medications for her heart were titrated down. It was astounding to the hospice team. They had never seen a hospice case improve so quickly. I was convinced it was all about what foods she ate and when she was putting them in her mouth. Hippocrates said, "Let your food be your medicine, and your medicine be your food."

As a child, I was lucky because we were fed very healthy foods. Later in life, I learned from decades of clinical experience how crucial it was for overall health and wellness to eat healthy foods.

When I was in private practice, I also had a second practice in a birthing center along with midwives, obstetricians, and pediatricians. By incorporating chiropractic care and medical prenatal care with a midwife, she and I pioneered a successful partnership of approaches that improved outcomes of pregnant women and babies. Our combined prenatal care reversed the threat of miscarriages, especially in mothers who became obese, threatening a gestational diabetic condition. Obese mothers develop extremely large babies which usually require a mandate for a C-section. Through short-term modification of the mother's diet by limiting starches and sugars with targeted nutritional supplementation, in the vast majorities of cases we had tremendous success with normalizing blood sugars and reducing the mother's weight to a level that prevented babies being large for their gestational age. The goal was to have a vaginal delivery naturally without drugs in the birth center or at home. The newborn then received a chiropractic adjustment and cranial manipulation to promote proper breastfeeding.

Globesity is something that can affect us from birth, and pretty much destroyed my family and caused us to watch the tortuous slow demise of my mother. When she became a prisoner in her body, it was felt by all of us around her. I realize now how sad I was.

Therefore, I am dedicating the last decades of my life to this cause because I have lived through the suffering and I have seen the broad damage of this condition. I pray that the FYF4Good Lifestyle resonates with the public, especially those who have tried everything, feel the decline of their health, and are feeling hopelessly out of control in this situation of obesity. We want to change the way that you look at food and give you control of your life to bring the freedom, peace of mind, happiness, self-esteem, and sense of well-being that the Higher Power has given us. We are healthy by design. FYF4Good is different, but not hard to master. You will eat for yourself to be lean and healthy 4Good, and you will NOT do it alone!

Victoria C. Arcadi DC DICCP is a Doctor of Chiropractic, with a Board Certified credential of Diplomate in Clinical Chiropractic Pediatrics, for licensed chiropractors in the specialty of pregnancy and pediatrics.

KATHLEEN J. POWELL

What Led Me to Flush Your Fat 4Good

It was a hot day in July 2015. I was thinking of the fun my sisters and I had growing up, convincing mom to let us turn on the lawn sprinklers, telling her it was so the grass would not die. What we really wanted was to put on our swimming suits and jump through the water. I was also thinking of my beautiful one-year-old god-daughter, Anja. Now I had a chance to relive this fun. She was going to have the best summer!

So I hopped into the car and headed to Target. I spent thirty minutes analyzing all of the options until I found the cutest little inflatable baby pool and a lawn sprinkler.

An hour later at their house, everything was perfect. The baby pool was filling up; the lawn sprinkler was running; I lined up the four little red wooden chairs that I had painted for her play room. These little chairs would give the whole family (Ma Ma, Da Da, Ah Ma (Chinese for Grandma) and Ka Ka (yes, that is what she calls me)) a way to join the fun.

Anja's mother brought her outside in the cutest little swimming suit: blue and white stripes with a red flower. Anja had just learned to walk so she was not about to sit still. Up and down, in and out, her face in the sprinkler, splashing water— it was constant movement. I sat as close as possible to her on that little red chair; wanting to soak in every moment of discovery and joy on her face.

But then I started feeling very sad. My thoughts went back to when I was a kid. I always wanted my mom to come outside and play in those sprinklers with us. I wanted her to jump in the hotel pool and play with me when we were on family vacations. But she was very overweight, obese actually, and I never saw her in a swimming suit. I knew she was too humiliated.

On that day in July, while watching Anja play, I realized I was at the heaviest weight of my adult life: 275 pounds and growing! I was depressed, sad, angry, humiliated (like my mom), hopeless, disappointed! You name a negative feeling, I probably felt it. I knew that the likelihood of seeing Anja graduate from college or get married and have children of her own was pretty close to zero. I was trying to be happy but was sad because I realized she would never see me in a swimming suit. I knew I would not take her swimming in a pool. No one was going to see my thighs! My attempt at making sure her childhood was filled with joy was becoming a torturous realization that I was not going to be in her life very long.

And then it happened; without warning. There was no loud sound. I did not hear the crack. Everything moved in slow motion. The world started to tilt. I was confused and dizzy. Was there an earthquake? Did I just have a stroke? Am I dying? Why was everyone standing now, with concerned looks on their faces, staring at me, but tilted?

Just than Anja's father came out of the house, glass of wine in hand, ready to join the *fun* and yelled: "What in the hell happened to the chair?" And then it hit me; the leg on the little red chair had broken and I was lying on the ground. My face turned bright red, and I wanted to cry.

The rest of the afternoon was a blur. I sat on a heavy-duty step stool from Home Depot while everyone else sat on the little red chairs. I felt like I was in time-out. I tried to laugh and have fun for Anja's sake, but the pain inside was too much.

I had tried just about every diet out there. A couple of times I was able to drop the weight, but if I wasn't sticking to baked chicken and brown rice, carefully measured, and a minimum of ninety minutes hard cardio *every day,* the weight would start to creep back up.

A few days after my humiliation by the baby pool, my phone rang. It was my sister, Jennifer. The sister, who rarely called, did. She wanted to tell me something before I came back to visit at the holidays (over five months away). I remember her saying it would not be fair to me if she did not share. *On and on* she went about these two amazing women she met, and how they knew so much about nutrition, and about a lifestyle she was learning. My sister normally didn't call me to share things going on in her life, so it was a strange call. I wanted her to get to the point so I could get off the phone and back to my self-misery.

Finally, I heard her say "In the last three months I have dropped thirty pounds. It is just melting off!" It was at that point I started to pay attention. You see, my sister was not going to be at the gym for three hours a day or starving herself thin. Had she gone mad? Had she joined a cult? She had never asked me to try anything like this before. Why should I listen to her about another fad diet? Oh, well. I had nothing to lose, and I felt I had lost my life already, so why not? At least I would be supporting my sister in the first thing that I had ever heard her speak this passionately about.

She told me what to do to get started and helped me with a shopping list. I only wanted to know the bare minimum. I did not want to invest any more time than was absolutely necessary if it wasn't going to work. But guess what? It did! The fat started burning off my body at the rate of three pounds a week. I couldn't believe it. How could this be true? Six months in and seventy-two pounds lighter, I had to know more, so I began to study it.

I decided I would write this book about the work of Jackie Padgette-Baird and Dr. Victoria Arcadi, not merely because I have lost over one hundred pounds following this Lifestyle, but because I saw my sister drop over ninety pounds and become a totally different person. Her personality changed. She became happy for the first time in her life! Her health drastically improved, and she was lean and fit and had amazing energy. And, surprisingly, she became a nicer person. We hadn't been close since grade school but are both having fun being sisters now.

Learning the Flush Your Fat 4Good Lifestyle was life changing! Not just because the fat burned off rapidly, but because it was *fun!* It changed everything I knew and felt about food and 'nutrifying' my body. It put me in control, and I continue to feel the health of my body improving every day. I want to share the Lifestyle that transformed my sister (and me).

In the United States alone there are over forty-five million people on a *diet* on any given day. Obesity is responsible for three hundred thousand (300,000) deaths every year in the United States, now the leading country in rates of obesity (percentage of the population that is obese). This is not only shocking, but totally unnecessary. I have a passion to see millions of lives changed, like my sister's, and like mine, through this journey! I hope you will join us.

What do you have to lose? ... besides the fat!

P.S. I now enjoy taking Anja to her weekly swim class and spending time swimming with her. Oh, what fun we have! Memories with Ka Ka that I know she will never forget.

SOURCES OF INFORMATION

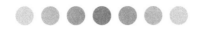

Airola, Paavo. *Every Woman's Book*. Arizona: Health Plus Publishers, 1979.

Allen, L.H. "How Common Is Vitamin B12 Deficiency?" *The American Journal of Clinical Nutrition* Vol 89: Issue 2: 693S-696S, February 2009.

American Heart Association Recommendations for Physical Activity in Adult. American Heart Association, July 27, 2016.

Anderson, W.A.D., Scotti, Thomas M. *Synopsis of Pathology, Tenth Edition.* Missouri: The C.V. Mosby Company, 1980.

Andrews, Ryan. "Phytates and Phytic Acid. Here's What You Need to Know." Precise Nutrition.com.

Angier, Natalie. "The Liver: A 'Blob' That Runs the Body." *The New York Times*, Health, June 12, 2017.

Artificial Sweeteners and Cancer. *National Institute of Cancer (NIH)*, August 10, 2016.

Balch, Phyllis A., CNC, Balch, James F., MD. *Nutritional Healing, Third Edition.* New York: Avery, 2000.

Banu, J., Bhattacharya, A., Rahman, M., Fernandes, G. "Beneficial Effects of Conjugated Linoleic Acid and Exercise on Bone of Middle-Aged Female Mice." *Journal of Bone and Mineral Metabolism* 26(5); (2008): 436-45. Epub 2008 Aug. 30.

Barker, Joel A. *Paradigms, The Business of Discovering the Future.* New York: HarperCollins Publishers Inc., 1992.

Behrman, Richard E. *Nelson Textbook of Pediatrics Fourteenth Edition.* Philadelphia: W.B. Saunders Company, 1992.

Bendtsen, L.Q., Lorenzen, J.K., Bendsen, N.T., Rasmussen, C., Astrup, A. "Effect of Dairy Proteins on Appetite Energy Expenditure, Body

Weight and Composition: A Review of the Evidence from Controlled Clinical Trials1." *Advances in Nutrition* (July 2013):Vol 3: 418-438.

"Black Currant Seed Oil." *Encyclopedia of Food Sciences and Nutrition*, Second Edition (2003).

Blank, Chris, *Proper Breathing Techniques for Walking.* Livingstrong.com (September 11, 2017).

Brodwin, Eric. "Most 'Biggest Loser' Winners Regain the Weight They Lost, and It Reveals a Disturbing Truth Behind Many Diets.*" Business Insider, Science* (May 2, 2016).

Carroll Aaron E. "Closest Thing to a Wonder Drug? Try Exercise.*" The New York Times* (June 20, 2016).

Chang J. and Kashyap, S. "The Protein-Sparing Modified Fast for Obese Patients with Type 2 Diabetes: What to Expect.*" Cleveland Clinic Journal of Medicine.* (2014 September) 81(9): 557-565.

Chaput, Jean-Phillipe. "Sleep Patterns, Diet Quality, and Energy Balance." *Physiology & Behavior,* 134 (July 2014): 86-91.

"Clinical Guidelines on the Identification, Evaluation and Treatment of Overweight and Obesity in Adults." *The Evidence Report, NIH Publication*, No. 98-4083, National Institutes of Health (September 1998).

Coldwell, Dr. Leonard. *Instinct Based Medicine: How to Survive Your Illness and Your Doctor.* New York: Strategic Book Publishing, 2008.

Copenhave, W. M., Johnson, D. D., *Bailey's Textbook of Histology*. Baltimore: The Williams & Wilkins Company, 1958.

Costantine, M. "Physiologic and Pharmacokinetic Changes in Pregnancy." *Frontiers in Pharacology 5* (2014): 65.

Crook, William G. *The Yeast Connection: A Medical Breakthrough*. Professional Books/Future Health, Incorporated, 1984.

"Dairy Products Inhibit Iron Absorption." *Articles, Conditions, Iron Deficiency Anemia, Nutrition,* July 13, 2014.

Davis, Margarett K., Isaacs, Charles E., Hanson, Lars A., Wright, Anne L. "Integrating Population Outcomes, Biological Mechanisms, and Research Methods in the Study of Human Milk and Lactation." Springer Science+Business Media, LLC.

DeCava, J. *The Real Truth About Vitamins and Antioxidants.* Columbus, Georgia: Brentwood Academic Press, 1996.

DelBrutto, O.H., Mera, R.M., Ha, J., Gillman, J., Zambrano, M., Castillo, P.R. "Dietary Fish Intake and Sleep Quality: A Population-Based Study." *Sleep Medicine*, Vol 17 (January 2016): 126-128.

Dries, Jan. *The Food Combining Bible*. Element, 2002.

Duffy, William. *Sugar Blues*. Warner Books by arrangement with Chilton Book Company, Chilton, PA, 1975.

Eaves, Ali. "Lifting Weights As You Age Cuts Your Risk of Early Death by 46: Discover the Science of How Strength Training Keeps You Young." *Men's Health* (March 23, 2016).

Edwards, S. "Sugar and the Brain." *On the Brain*. The Harvard Mahoney Neuroscience Institute Letter.

Ferdman, Roberto. "Why Diets Actually Don't Work According to a Researcher Who Has Studied Them for Decades." *The Washington Post*, May 4, 2015.

Field, C.J., Schley, P.D. "Evidence for Potential Mechanisms for the Effect of Conjugated Linoleic Acid on Tumor Metabolism and Immune Function: Lessons from n-3 Fatty Acids1'2'3'4." *The American Journal of Clinical Nutrition*, 2004.

"2017 Framingham Heart Study." A Project of the National Heart, Lung, and Blood Institute at Boston University.

Gebel, K., Ding, D., Chey, T., Stamatakis, E., Brown, W.J., Bauman, A.E., "Effect of Moderate to Vigorous Physical Activity on All-Cause Mortality in Middle-Aged and Older Australians." *JAMA Internal Medicine* 175(6). (June 2015): 970-7.

GMO FAQ, *"Where are GMOs Grown and Banned?"* Genetic Literacy Project, Science Trumps Ideology.

Gormley, James J. *DHA: A Good Fat Essential for Life*. New York: Kensington Publishing Corp., 1999.

Gray, Henry. *Gray's Anatomy*. New York: Bounty Books, 1977.

Guyton, Arthur C., *Function of the Human Body, Fourth Edition*. Philadelphia: W.B. Saunders Company, 1974.

Guyton, Arthur C., *Textbook of Medical Physiology 5th Edition*. Philadelphia: W.B. Saunders, 1976.

Hartmann, E. "Effects of L-Tryptophan on Sleepiness and on Sleep." *Journal of Psychiatric Research* 17(2) (1982-83): 107-113.

Hay, William H. M.D. *Health via Food*. Soil and Health Library, 1929.

Hur, A.J., Park, Y. "Effect of Conjugated Linoleic Acid on Bone Formation and Rheumatoid Arthritis." *European Journal of Pharmacology*. 568(1–3); (2007 Jul 30):16–24. Epub 2007 May 22.

Hussein G., Nakagawa T., Goo, H., Shimada Y., Matsumoto, K., Sankawa, U., Watanabe, H., "Astaxanthin Ameliorates Features of Metabolic Syndrome." *Life Sciences*, 80(6); (Jan. 16 2007): 522–9. Epub 2006 Oct 12.

Jacob, Stanley W., MD, F.A.C.S. *Structure and Function in Man*. Philadelphia, London, Toronto: W.B Saunders Company, 1970.

Joklik, W. K., Willett, H.P., Amos, D. B., *17th Edition, Zinsser Microbiology*. New York: Appleton-Century-Crofts, 1980.

Joklik, Wolfgang K., Willet, Hilda P., Amos, D. Bernard, *Zinsser Microbiology, 17th Edition*. New York: Appleton-Century-Crofts, 1980.

Jurgonski A., Fotschki B., Juskiewicz, J. "Disparate Metabolic Effects of Black Currant Seed Oil in Rats Fed a Basal and Obesogenic Diet." *European Journal of Nutrition*, 54(6); (2015: 991–999.

Karger, L. *ActaAnatomica*. Basel, Freiburg, Paris, London, New York, New Delhi, Bangkok, Singapore, Tokyo, Sydney: Medical and Scientific Publishers, 1998.

Kempner W., Newborg B.C., Peschel R.L, Skyler, J.S. "Treatment of Massive Obesity with Rice/Reduction Diet Program. An Analysis of 106 Patients with at Least a 45-Kg Weight Loss." *Arch Intern Med*. (1975 Dec);135(12):1575–84.

Kennedy, A., Martinez, K., Schmidt, S., Mandrup, S., LaPoint, K., McIntosh, M. "Antiobesity Mechanisms of Action of Conjugated Linoleic Acid." *The Journal of Nutritional Biochemistry*, 21(3); (2010 Mar): 171–179.

Kennedy, David. *How to Save Your Teeth, Toxic-Free Preventive Dentistry*. Health Action Press, Ohio, 1993.

"Ketones." Diabetes Education Online, Diabetes Teaching Center at the University of California, San Francisco.

Kibangou, I.B., et al. "Milk Proteins and Iron Absorption: Contrasting Effects of Different Caseinophosphopeptides." *Pediatric Research*. 2005.

Kirschmann, John D., Dunne, Lavon J. *Nutriton Almanac*, Second Edition. McGraw Hill paperback edition, 1984.

Kishimoto, Y., Yoshida H., Kondo K. "Potential Anti-Atherosclerotic Properties of Astaxanthin." *Mar Drugs*. (2016 Feb); 14(2): 35.

Krause, Marie V., Mahan, Kathleen L. *Food, Nutrition, and Diet Therapy*. Philadelphia, London, Toronto: W.B. Sounders Company, 1979.

Krebs, N., Himes, J., Jacobson, D., Nicklas, T., Guilday, P., Styne, D. "Assessment of Child and Adolescent Overweight and Obesity." *Journal of Pediatrics* (2007): 120:S193-S228.

Langman, Jan. *Medical Embryology, Third Edition*. Baltimore: Williams & Wilkins, 1975.

Layman, D.K., Evans, E.M., Erickson, D., Seyler, J., Weber, J., Bagshaw, D., Griel, A., Psota, T., Kris Etherton, P. "A Moderate-Protein Diet Produces Sustained Weight Loss and Long-Term Changes in Body Composition and Blood Lipids in Obese Adults 1, 2." *The Journal of Nitrition*, Vol 139 No. 3 (Jan 21, 2009): 514-521.

Layman, D.K., Evans, E., Baum, J.I., Seyler, J., Erickson, D.J., Boileau, R.A., "Dietary Protein and Exercise Have Additive Effects on Body Composition During Weight Loss in Adult Women 1, 2." *The Journal of Nitrition*, Vol 135 No.8 (Aug 1, 2005): 1903-1910.

Lee, Bruce Y. "*Global Obesity Epidemic: New Studies Show How Big a Problem It's Become*." *Forbes Pharma & Healthcare/#PublicHealth*, June 13, 2017.

Leidy, H.J., Clifton, P.M., Astrup, A., Wycherley, T.P., Westerterp-Plantenga, M.S., Luscombe-Marsh, N.D., Woods, S.C., Mattes, R.D. "The Role of Protein in Weight Loss and Maintenance 1,2,3,4,5." *The American Journal of Clinical Nutrition* Vol 101 No. 6 (June 2015): 1320S-1329S.

Lifshitz, F., et al. "Globesity: The Root Causes of the Obesity Epidemic in the USA and Now Worldwide." *Pediatric Endocrinology Reviews*, 2014.

Li J., Zhang, N., Hu, L., Li, Z., Li, R., Li, C., Wang, S. "Improvement in Chewing Activity Reduces Energy Intake in One Meal and Modulates Plasma Gut Hormone Concentrations in Obese and Lean Young Chinese Men." *The American Journal of Clinical Nutrition* 94(3); (September, 2011): 709-16. Doi: 10.3945/ajcn. 111.015164. Epub 2011 Jul 20.

Lipton, Bruce, *The Biology of Belief: Unleashing the Power of Consciousness, Matter, & Miracles*. California: Mountain of Love/Elite Books, 2005.

Longland, T.M., Oikawa, S.Y., Mitchell, C.J., Devries, M.C., Phillips, S.M. "Higher Compared with Lower Dietary Protein During an Energy Deficit Combined with Intense Exercise Promotes Greater Lean Mass Gain and Fat Mass Loss: A Randomized Trial 1,2." *The American Journal of Clinical Nutrition,* December 16, 2015.

Lopez, B.G., Bacardi, G.M., DE, Lira, G.C., Jimenez, C.A., "Meal Replacement Efficacy on Long-Term Weight Loss: A Systemic Review." *Nutricion Hospitalaria* 26(6); (2011 Nov.-Dec.): 1260-5.

Luce, Gay G., *Body Time: Physiological Rhythms and Stress.* New York: Pantheon, 1971.

Luce, Gay G., Segal, J., *Slep.* Coward-McCann, 1966.

Ma, G., et al. "Phytate Intake and Molar Ratios of Phytate to Zinc, Iron and Calcium in the Diets of People in China." *European Journal of Clinical Nutrition* 61 (2007): 368-374.

Mendelsohn, Robert S., *Confessions of a Medical Heretic.* New York: Warner Books, 1980.

Modan, M.H., Halkin, S., Almoz, A., Lusky, A., Eshkol, M., Sketi, A., Sdetra and Z. Fuchs, "Hyperinsulinemia: A link Between Hypertension, Obesity and Glucose Intolerance," *Journal of Clinical Investigation* 75 (1985): 809-817.

Mondoa, Emil I., *Sugars That Heal: The New Healing Science of Glyconutrients.* New York: The Ballantine Publishing Group, 2001.

Moore, S.C., Lee, M., Weiderpass, E, et al. "Association of Leisure-Time Physical Activity with Risk of 26 Types of Cancer in 1.44 Million Adults. *JAMA Internal Medicine* 176(6); (2016): 816-825.

Munro, H.N., et al. *Mammalian Protein Metabolism.* New York: Academic Press, 1970.

Murray, Robert K. In *Harpers Biochemistry, 24th Edition*, Chapter 56: 646. Connecticut: Appleton & Lange, 1996.

Noakes, T.D. "Low-Carbohydrate and High-Fat Intake Can Manage Obesity and Associated Conditions: Occasional Survey." *South Africa Medical Journal* 103 (2013):824–825. doi: 10.7196/samj.7343.

Null, Ga. *Food Combining Handbook.* New York: Jove, 1981.

OECD (Organization for Economic Cooperation and Development) Obesity Update 2017.

Palgi, A., Read, J. L., Greenberg, M., Hoefer, M. A., Bistrian. B. R., Black-burn. G. L.

"Multidisciplinary Treatment of Obesity with a Protein-Sparing Modi-fied Fast: Results in 668 Outpatients." *American Journal of Public Health* 75(10); (1985): 1190-1194.

Park, J.S., Chyun, J.H., Kim, K.Y., Line, L.L., Chew, B.P. "Astaxanthin Decreased Oxidative Stress and Inflammation Enhanced Immune Response in Humans." *Nutrition & Metabolism* 2010.

Pavlov, Ivan P. *The Work of the Digestive Glands.* London: Griffin, 1902.

Payton, Matt. "*A New Study Claims That Sugar Has the Same Effect on the Brain As Cocaine.*" *The Independent,* April 13, 2016.

Peth, J.A., Kinnick. T.R., Youngblood, E.B., Tritschler, H.J., Henriksen, E. J. "Effects of a Unique Conjugate of Alpha-Lipoic Acid and Gamma-Linolenic Acid on Insulin Action in Obese Zucker Rats." *American Jour-nal of Physiology-Regulatory Ingegrative and Comparative Physiology* 278(2); (2000 Feb.):: R453-9.

Peuhkuri, K., Shivola, N., Korpela, R. "Diet Promotes Sleep Duration." *Nutrition Research* 32(5); (2012), 309-319.

Phinney, S.D., Tang, A.B., Thurmond, D.C., Nakamura, M.T., Stern, J.S. "Abnormal Polyunsaturated Lipid Metabolism in the Obese Zucker Rat, with Partial Metabolic Correction by Gamma-Linolenic Acid Administration. *Metabolism* 42(9); (1993): 1127-1140.

Phinney, Stephen. *The Art and Science of Nutritional Ketosis.* University of California, San Francisco: Advancing Health Worldwide presentation, November 16, 2012.

Lecture by Dr. Stephen D. Phinney. "The Case for Nutritional Ketosis."

Price, Weston A., DDS, *Nutrition and Physical Degeneration.* Price-Pottenger, 1939.

Qipshidze-Kelm, N., Kellianne, M.P., Solinger, J.C., Cole, M.P. "Co-Treatment With Conjugated Linoleic Acid And Nitrite Protects Against Myocardial Infarction. *Redox Biology* Volume 2, (2014), 1-7.

Rabinowitz, D. and K.L. Zierler, "Forearm Metabolism in Obesity and Its Response to Intra-Arterial Insulin, Chariacterizaton of Insulin Resis-tance and Evidence for Adaptive Hyperinsulinism," *Journal of Clinical Investigation* 41 (1962): 2173-2181.

Reynolds, Gretchen. "A Diet and Exercise Plan to Lose Weight and Gain Muscle." *The New York Times*, February 3, 2016.

Reynolds, Gretchen. "Ask Well: The 10-20-30 Workout for Swimmers. *The New York Times*, January 22, 2016.

Reynolds, Gretchen. "Benefits of Exercise Diminish After Short Rest." *The New York Times*, September 28, 2016.

Reynolds, Gretchen. "Exercise Tied to Lower Risk for 13 Types of Cancer." *The New York Times*, Mary 18, 2016.

Reynolds, Gretchen. "Lifting Lighter Weights Can Be Just as Effective as Heavy Ones." *The New York Times*, July 20, 2016.

Reynolds, Gretchen. "The Right Dose of Exercise for a Longer Life." *The New York Times*, April 15, 2015.

Reynolds, Gretchen. "Which Type of Exercise Is Best for the Brain? *The New York Times*, February 17, 2016.

Reynolds, Gretchen. "Why Exercise Is Good for the Heart." *The New York Times*, February 15, 2017.

Riserus, U., Berglund, L., Vessby, B. "Conjugated Linoleic Acid (CLA) Reduced Abdominal Adipose Tissue in Obese Middle-Aged Men with Signs of the Metabolic Syndrome: A Randomized Controlled Trial." *International Journal of Obesity* 25 (2001): 1129-1135.

Robbins, Stanley L, Cotran, Ramzi S., *Pathologic Basis of Disease, Second Edition*. Philadelphia: W.B. Saunders Company, 1979.

Schirmer, M.A., Phinney, S.D. "Gamma-Linolenate Reduces Weight Regain in Formerly Obese Humans." *The Journal of Nutrition* 137(6); (2007): 1430-5.

Schlachter, M., MD, Aristotle, T., D.C., L.Ac., *In Search of Manna*. Las Vegas, Nevada: Sano Press, 2003.

Schlemmer, U, et al. "Phytate in Foods and Significance for Humans: Food Sources, Intake Processing, Bioavailability, Protective Role and Analysis." *Molecular Nutrition & Food Research* 53 (2009): S330-S375.

Seim, H.C., Rigden, S.R. "Approaching the Protein-Sparing Modified Fast." *American Family Physician*. (1990 Nov: 42(5 Suppl): 51S-56S.

Schmidt, M.A. *Childhood Ear Infections*. California: North Atlantic Books, 1990.

Schmidt, M.A. *Smart Fats, How Dietary Fats and Oils Affect Mental, Physical and Emotional Intelligence*. Berkeley, California: Frog Limited, 1997.

Shelton, Herbert M. *Dr. Shelton's Hygienic Review, Volume 3 1941-1942.* Health Research 1996.

Shelton, Herbert M. *Exercise.* Chicago: Natural Hygiene Press, 1971.

Shelton, Herbert M. *Fasting Can Save Your Life.* Chicago: Natural Hygiene Press, 1964.

Shelton, Herbert M. *Food Combining Made Easy.* Dr. Shelton's Health School, Texas 1951.

Shelton, Herbert M. *Food Combining Made Easy.* Willow Pub, Texas, 1982.

Shelton, Herbert M. *Food Combining Made Easy, 3rd Edition.* Book Publishing Company, 2011.

Shelton, Herbert M. *Principles of Natural Hygiene.* Dr. Shelton's Health School, Texas 1964.

Shelton, Herbert M. "The Digestion of Milk." *Hygiene Review*, August 1969.

Shelton, Herbert M. *The Hygiene Care of Children.* Connecticut: Natural Hygiene Press, 1981.

Shelton, Herbert M. *The Hygiene System*, Vol. I, II & III, Dr. Shelton's Health School, Texas, 1934.

Smith, Lendon H., *Feed Your Body Right, Understanding Your Individual Body Chemistry For Proper Nutrition Without Guesswork*, M. Evans and Company, Inc., New York (1994).

Smith, Lendon H. *How to Raise A Healthy Child.* New York: M. Evans and Company, Inc., 1996.

Soma-Pillay P., Nelson-Piercy, C., Tolppanen, H. Mebazaa A. "Physiological Changes in Pregnancy." *Cardiovascular Journal of Africa* 27(2); (2016 March-April): 89-94.

Spencer, R. P. *The Intestinal Tract.* Illinois: Charles Thomas Publishers, 1960.

Somersall, Allan C. *The Healing Power of 8 Sugars.* Canada: The Natural Wellness Group, 2005.

Steck, S.E., Chalecki, A.M., Miller, P., Conway, J., Austin, G.L., Hardin, J.W., Albright, C.D., Thuillier, P. "Conjugated Linoleic Acid Supplementation for Twelve Weeks Increases Lean Body Mass in Obese Humans." *The Journal of Nutrition* 137(5); (2007 May): 1189-93.

Stoff, Jesse A., Pellegrino, Charles R. *Chronic Fatigue Syndrome: The Hidden Epidemic.* New York: Random House, 1988.

Takahashi, Y., Ide, T., Fujita, H. "Dietary Gamma-Linolenic Acid in the Form of Borage Oil Causes Less Body Fat Accumulation Accompanying an Increase in Uncoupling Protein 1 Mrna Level In Brown Adipose Tissue." *Comparative Biochemistry and Physiology Part B: Biochemistry and Molecular Biology* 127(2): (2000 Oct.): 213-22.

The GBD 2015 Obesity Collaborators. "Health Effects of Overweight and Obesity in 195 Countries over 25 Years." *New England Journal of Medicine* 377 (2017): 13-27.

The International College of Applied Nutrition. *Nutrition-Applied Personally*. LaHabra, California: International College of Applied Nutrition, 1973.

"The Power of Natural Astaxanthin for Increased Muscle Performance." *Nutraceutical Business Review*, August 15, 2014.

Thiel, Robert. *The Truth About Vitamins in Nutritional Supplements*. Doctors' Research, Inc.

Thurmond D.C., Tang, A.B., Nakamura, M.T., Stern, J.S., Phinney, S.D. "Time-Dependent Effects Of Progressive Gamma-Linolenate Feeding On Hyperphagia, Weight Gain, And Erythrocyte Fatty Acid Composition During Growth Of Zucker Obese Rats." *Obesity Reearch & Clinical Practice* 1(2); (1993 March): 118-25.

Trowbridge, John P. and Walker, Morton *The Yeast Syndrome: How to Help Your Doctor Identify and Treat The Real Cause of Your Yeast-Related Illness*. United States and Canada: Random House Publishing Group, 1986.

Understanding Childhood Obesity, *American Heart Association*, 2010.

University of Maryland Medical Center. Gamma-Linolenic Acid, Overview, 2017.

U.S. Department of Health and Human Sciences, (NIH) National Institute of Diabetes and Digestive and Kidney Disease. *Nonalcoholic Fatty Liver Disease & NASH*, November 2016.

Varki, A., Cummings, R., Esko, J., Hart, G., Marth, J. *Essentials of Glycobiology*. New York: Cold Spring Harbor Laboratory Press, 1999.

Vohra, A., Satyanarayana, T. "Phytases: Microbal Sources, Production, Purification and Potential Biotechnological Applications." *Critical Reviews in Biotechnology*. (2003;23): 29-60.

Volek, J.S., PhD, R.D., Jeff, S. Phinney, M.D., PhD, Stephen, D. "The Art and Science of Low Carbohydrate Living," Beyond Obesity, LLC, 2011.

Volek, JS., Phinney, SD. *The Art and Science of Low Carbohydrate Performance.* Beyond Obesity LLC; 2012.

Volek J.S., Freidenreich D.J., Saenz, C., Kunces, L.J., Creighton, B.C., Bartley, J.M., Davitt, P.M., Munoz, C.X., Anderson, J.M., Maresh, C.M., Lee, E.C., Schuenke. M.D., Aemi. G., Kraemer, W.J., Phinney, S.D. "Metabolic Characteristics of Keto-Adapted Ultra-Endurance Runners," *Metabolism,* Vol 65, Issue 3 (March 2016), 100-110.

Waerland, Are. *Health Is Your Birthright.* Switzerland: Humata Publishers, Circa 1945.

Waerland, Ebba. *Cancer: A Disease of Civilization.* Ontario Canada: Provoker Press, 1980.

Walker, Matthew. *Why We Sleep, Unlocking the Power of Sleep and Dreams,* Scribner, Imprint of Simon and Schuster Inc., October 2017.

Walther, David S. *Applied Kinesiology, Volume II.* Colorado: Systems DC, 1983.

Webb, Nicholas J. *The Cost of Being Sick: Surviving the Healthcare Meltdown,* 2nd Edition. Orem, Utah: Sound Concepts, Inc., 2003.

"Whole Milk Linked with Cancer." *Nutritional Health Review,* 1983.

Wigmore, Ann. *Be Your Own Doctor.* Boston: Hippocrates Health Institute, 1973.

Williams, Roger J. *The Wonderful World Within You.* Kansas: Biocomunications Press, 1987.

Wing, R., Lang, W., Wadden, T., Safford, M., Knowler, W., Bertoni, A., Hill, J., Brancati, F., Peters, A., Wagenknecht, L. Look AHEAD Research Group. "Benefits of Modest Weight Loss in Improving Cardiovascular Risk Factors in Overweight and Obese Individuals with Type 2 Diabetes." *Diabetes Care.* (2011 Jul, 34(7): 1481-1486.

Winter, Ruth. *Beware of the Food You Eat.* New York: Signet, 1971.

Wyngaarden, James B., Smith, Lloyd H. *Cecil Textbook of Medicine, 17th Edition.* Philadelphia: W.B. Saunders Company, 1985.

Yahia, Elhadi M. *Fruit and Vegetable Phytochemicals: Chemistry and Human Health (2 Volumes).* John Wiley & Sons, August 25, 2017.

Yeonhwa P., Albright K.J., Liu W., Storckson, J.M., Cook, M.E., Pariza, M.W. "Effect Of Conjugated Linoleic Acid on Body Composistion in Mice. *Lipids* Volume 32, Issue 8 (August 1997): 853-858.

Younossi Z., Anstee, Q.M., Marietti, M., Hardy, T., Henry, L., Eslam, M., Bugianesi, J.G., Bugianesi, E. "Global burden of NAFLD and NASH: Trends, Predictions, Risk Factors and Prevention." *Nature Reviews Gastroenterology & Hepatology*, (2018): 15, 11-20.